AF806170

The Palgrave Lacan Series

Series Editors
Calum Neill
Edinburgh Napier University
Edinburgh, UK

Derek Hook
Duquesne University
Pittsburgh, USA

Jacques Lacan is one of the most important and influential thinkers of the 20th century. The reach of this influence continues to grow as we settle into the 21st century, the resonance of Lacan's thought arguably only beginning now to be properly felt, both in terms of its application to clinical matters and in its application to a range of human activities and interests. The Palgrave Lacan Series is a book series for the best new writing in the Lacanian field, giving voice to the leading writers of a new generation of Lacanian thought. The series will comprise original monographs and thematic, multi-authored collections. The books in the series will explore aspects of Lacan's theory from new perspectives and with original insights. There will be books focused on particular areas of or issues in clinical work. There will be books focused on applying Lacanian theory to areas and issues beyond the clinic, to matters of society, politics, the arts and culture. Each book, whatever its particular concern, will work to expand our understanding of Lacan's theory and its value in the 21st century.

Nick Stock • Nick Peim

The Lacanian Teacher

Education, Pedagogy and Enjoyment

palgrave
macmillan

Nick Stock
Education and Social Justice
University of Birmingham
Birmingham, UK

Nick Peim
Education and Social Justice
University of Birmingham (retired)
Birmingham, UK

ISSN 2946-4196 ISSN 2946-420X (electronic)
The Palgrave Lacan Series
ISBN 978-3-031-93017-1 ISBN 978-3-031-93018-8 (eBook)
https://doi.org/10.1007/978-3-031-93018-8

© The Editor(s) (if applicable) and The Author(s), under exclusive license to Springer Nature Switzerland AG 2025

This work is subject to copyright. All rights are solely and exclusively licensed by the Publisher, whether the whole or part of the material is concerned, specifically the rights of translation, reprinting, reuse of illustrations, recitation, broadcasting, reproduction on microfilms or in any other physical way, and transmission or information storage and retrieval, electronic adaptation, computer software, or by similar or dissimilar methodology now known or hereafter developed.
The use of general descriptive names, registered names, trademarks, service marks, etc. in this publication does not imply, even in the absence of a specific statement, that such names are exempt from the relevant protective laws and regulations and therefore free for general use.
The publisher, the authors and the editors are safe to assume that the advice and information in this book are believed to be true and accurate at the date of publication. Neither the publisher nor the authors or the editors give a warranty, expressed or implied, with respect to the material contained herein or for any errors or omissions that may have been made. The publisher remains neutral with regard to jurisdictional claims in published maps and institutional affiliations.

Cover illustration: duncan1890

This Palgrave Macmillan imprint is published by the registered company Springer Nature Switzerland AG.
The registered company address is: Gewerbestrasse 11, 6330 Cham, Switzerland

If disposing of this product, please recycle the paper.

To Martha

Acknowledgements

Nick Stock would like to thank the British Academy for their fellowship funding, allowing me to complete this book. He would also like to thank his colleagues at the University of Birmingham, especially Ian McGimpsey. These colleagues gave feedback in talks and conversations concerning some of the topics in this book. He wants to give special mention to his Psychoanalytic Society, a group he ran whilst teaching in a college. They regularly contributed educational examples to elucidate the concepts being explored in the set psychoanalytic reading (and demonstrated that you *can* give Freud and Lacan to teenagers). He especially wants to thank his wife Sarah who supported him in finishing the book, particularly during the long evenings of editing. Finally, he extends sincere thanks to his friend and mentor Nick Peim, without whom he never could have written this book.

Nick Peim would like to thank Nick Stock who not only conceived of this book but who also steered its progress and whose friendship has been a rich pedagogical dividend. He would also like to pay tribute to the memory of Paul Moran, 'il miglior fabbro', whose faith in my interest in Lacan long ago sustained my troubled reading in psychoanalysis. Let me also give special thanks to Elizabeth, Kate, Louise, and James who, among others, continue to 'make life worth living'.

Contents

1 Approaching Education with Lacan 1

2 The Teacher 29

3 Fantasies of Teaching 55

4 On the Structures of Pedagogy 93

5 The Impossibility of Pedagogical Alternatives 127

6 The Jouissance of Teaching 147

Glossary 189

References 199

Index 201

List of Abbreviations

1. Citations from Freud's papers will be marked by the letters SE (standing for "Standard Edition") followed by a volume number in Roman numerals and a page number: (SE II, p.100)

Example: Freud, S. (1895). *The Standard Edition of the Complete Psychological Works of Sigmund Freud, Volume II (1893–1895): Studies on Hysteria*. The Hogarth Press.

2. Citations from Lacan's published seminars will be marked by their number in Roman numerals and a page number: (VII, p.100)

Example: Lacan, J. (2008). *The Ethics of Psychoanalysis. The Seminars of Jacques Lacan: Book VII*. Routledge.

3. Citations from Lacan's writings will be marked by the abbreviation of their title and page number: (E, p.330)

Example: Lacan, J. (2006). *Écrits* (B. Fink, Trans.). W.W. Norton and Co.

CHAPTER 1

Approaching Education with Lacan

Abstract Beginning with commonplace, empirical accounts of teachers' motivation, the chapter considers the potency of Lacanian psychoanalysis in approaching the discourses of education that shape the teacher's self-image. The relations between psychoanalysis, Lacan and teaching are then touched on with some reference to Lacan's seminars, asking the question of why psychoanalysis is necessary for thinking about education and why it is so commonly disavowed. The philosophical threads of Lacan's thought are explored in their relation to the orders of education. Lacanian ontology is explored in its relation to the world of education and the specific institution of the school, drawing on the intersecting registers of the Real, Symbolic and Imaginary.

Keywords Real • Symbolic • Imaginary • Ontology • Freud • Philosophy of Education • School • Teaching

...we place no trust in altruistic feeling, we who lay bare the aggressivity that underlies the activity of the philanthropist, the idealist, the pedagogue, and even the reformer.
*—Jacques Lacan (*Écrits*, p. 81)*

© The Author(s), under exclusive license to Springer Nature Switzerland AG 2025

N. Stock, N. Peim, *The Lacanian Teacher*, The Palgrave Lacan Series, https://doi.org/10.1007/978-3-031-93018-8_1

My Teaching

If you ask a teacher why they got into teaching, you might hear an eerily repetitious response. They are likely to enunciate a predictable set of desires, usually bound to salvific and redemptive subject positions. 'Making a difference', 'helping others', 'guiding children', 'giving them a better future'. Lacan recognises the sickness in these sorts of desires, 'the aggressivity that underlies the activity of the philanthropist, the idealist, the pedagogue, and even the reformer' (E, p. 81). From this point of view, redemptive desire is always-already coupled with the horror of its death drive, its aggression, and its ceaseless pursuit of enjoyment. There is, thus, something unsettling and perverse about the desire of the teacher, and something we should be concerned by when we take the logics of education as they are always presented to us: as inherently good. The purely positive orientation of education is disturbed by any serious Lacanian account.

But teachers often do something else curiously clinical that many other professions do not when you ask them about their jobs. They recount a 'primal scene' retroactively identified as the moment they knew they wanted to be a teacher. Often, it involves a singular teacher and a singular classroom moment, some great unveiling of a text, concept, or idea. In fantasmatic language, the teacher recounts the Other that they wished to become, so they too could recreate these uncanny moments. The through-line from these scenes to teaching are clear so that the teacher as figure in the domain of the school may confidently begin to construct their own meaningful narrative of the self. Teachers thus seem to know not only what they are doing and who they do it for, but why they do it too.

We are less certain. The integrity of such narratives is problematized by the fantasies they harbour. Even so, the authors of this book are not unaffected by the lure of the redemptive desires of teaching. Both, though in very different decades, started their careers as a teacher of English in Secondary Schools in the UK, teaching students up to the age of 18 about Shakespeare, Romanticism, Modernism, writing, verse, and so on. After some time in this position, both left teaching to work in a university. One took a detour to train English teachers, but both eventually ended up researching education and of course continued to teach in seminars and lectures. Much of what we discuss in the book recalls examples or cites images of teaching, usually (but not always) from the high school English Literature classroom. We too were English teachers with some emphasis on nurturing creativity and growth through language use, after all. But 'the English teacher' in itself is an important figure in the fantasies of education. As we raise in Chap. 3, most depictions of teachers in films and literature feature an English teacher. As a figure, it encapsulates the most powerful and life-changing educator there is, one whose lessons are contentless in terms of fixed knowledge, but imagined as radically enlightening in the inherent process of guiding students through reading and thinking. In this way, the English teacher stands as the fantasmatic educator *par excellence*. We think examples of English teaching encapsulate much of what teaching is imagined to be writ large, a position of the altruist, the ur-pedagogue, the one always 'making a difference', 'helping others', 'guiding children', and 'offering them a better future'.

The use of the signifier 'education' here is not accidental and not to be confused with the common criticism of the school and schooling. There is a critical stance towards the school common in academic circles that touches on the story of education in modernity. It is not uncommon to see educationalists expound a fatal deconstruction of schooling only to uphold the concept, the *fantasy* even, of 'education' as a transcendental good that can, one fine day, be fully materialised. But the very act of the materialisation of education shapes itself as the school as we know it. It is a bringing forth from the Symbolic, the name Lacan gives to the linguistic structure of our world. The school, we claim, is the key instrument of governance in modernity, the paradigm institution of education that other institutions (universities, nurseries) are ontologically congruent with. We might also add, as Lacan might say, schools constitute a vital signifier in the Symbolic order of education. Indeed, what we have sought to reveal previously in our work is the fantasmatic dimension of education that pervades its Symbolic structure. As educators 'we'—the teachers, researchers, and students—must reside within this structure of fantasy that entails redemption, egalitarianism, meritocracy, even blunt utilitarian functionalism for all those that would take part in its mission, a structure of fantasy we will explore further. We hover between various fantasies as teachers, including the fantasy of the hopeless condition of youth, culture, world, curriculum, comprehensive school, and so forth; such images may promote the unconscious trace that education might be irredeemable despite all best efforts to research, improve, reform and troubleshoot. We have previously made the irony of this clear, that we are only ever taking this stance from the inside of education, that we too are complicit in its

Symbolic function, that we cannot go beyond the order of education that we write and work within: 'no metalanguage can be spoken' (E, p. 688).

From a consideration of the disjunction between educational fantasies and realities hovers the haunting presence of another question. In one author's PhD viva, ironically another Symbolic space of education, an examiner asked how, despite the eighty thousand words or so of deconstruction of education and redescription of it as a monstrosity, you still teach in a school; why do that? Presuming a necessary ethical dimension in being a teacher, the question '*How* can you do that if there is nothing redeemable about education?' suggests incredulity. I was surely aware of my place within this horrifying picture that I had laid bare, and yet somehow could find it within myself to go on teaching. The question of *my teaching* became central, and the only answer that I mustered was, well, 'I enjoy it'. Enjoyment, *jouissance* as Lacan names it, both its pleasures and its pains, left only one place to turn. It is with this question of enjoyment that we as teachers and educational researchers felt we must turn, or *return*, to psychoanalysis.

The question of teaching for the teacher is shared by the authors and the French psychoanalyst Jacques Lacan, a figure who offers the possibility of the exploration taking place in this book. The Lacanian teacher, as we coin in the book's title, is the (often reluctant) teacher who was Jacques Lacan, and the teacher who takes account of Lacan's ideas. Lacan is invoked both materially and to name a way of thinking that is appropriately philosophical for the condition of our times. It is only through occupying the space of these different figures of Lacan that we have been able to do justice to the question of 'my teaching'. We thus explore the direct and passing references that Lacan himself makes to teaching, entailing a consideration of *how* Lacan taught in the manner of his speech, his preference for speech over writing, the logics of his pedagogy, and his attempts at forming both a psychoanalytic school and educational groups in the form of 'the cartels'.[1] But the other angle that we will take is exploring how Lacan's key ideas can help us rethink what it means to be a teacher in the educational landscape of the contemporary moment and beyond. This is not a manifesto positing that teachers should aim to be more like

[1]We are not the first to attend to such a task. The lecture given by Dany Nobus (19th November, 2023) to the *Lacan Salon* is a particularly pertinent biographical examination of Lacan's teaching, and indeed others (Felman, 1982; Ellsworth, 1997; Roseboro, 2008; Webster, 2023) have done similar work.

psychoanalysts, though as Lacan makes clear, there are lessons to be learned from the position of the analyst for the position of teaching. Rather, echoing and going beyond the work of Britzman, Ellsworth and Felman, we are interested in what we might learn (if such a thing can even occur) from psychoanalytic logic to bring into the classroom. This is not just a transposition: though psychoanalysis is a discipline predicated on its place within a clinical encounter between analyst and analysand, we find resonance between this space and the space of the classroom in a way that is not found readily in other environments. If we think of the psychoanalytic space that Lacan dedicates his career to as an intimate encounter between one and another, where questions of desire, knowledge, fantasy, identification, and repression occur, we could just as easily say that this is the space of the classroom too. Psychoanalysis as a mode of thinking and relationality, not a body of knowledge, offers a major contribution to educational thought that remains generally unmined.

It is surprising that Lacanian thought has not fully penetrated the sphere of education. Right from the opening of Lacan's first seminar in 1953 there is an allusion to and destabilising of the teacher:

> The master breaks the silence with anything—with a sarcastic remark, with a kick-start. That is how a Buddhist master conducts his search for meaning, according to the technique of zen. It beseeches students to find out for themselves the answer to their own questions. The master does not teach *ex cathedra* a readymade science; he supplies an answer when the students are on the verge of finding it. (I, p. 1)

The position of mastery held by the figure of teacher is called into question, with an overturning of knowledge to the student, but coupled with a Symbolic power held by the teacher through their acts. It is not the sharing of knowledge in a teaching relationship that Lacan praises here, but an interjection of a signifier to propel the student into a search for their own answers. Still, this sort of educational perspective is not that different from various schools of pedagogy, critical or not. As Lacan's career goes on, a career dominated by teaching, his educational perspectives become more radical and unique.

In 1967, Lacan gave a short lecture at an asylum in Lyon which he titled *The Place, Origin and End of My Teaching*. Less trenchant than Lacan's twenty-five seminars or the *Écrits,* nevertheless there is an important aspect of Lacan's thinking at the forefront of this talk. It is here that Lacan refers to his position as a teacher, as one that we may imagine transmits knowledge to an audience of learners (something he will problematise again and again). Lacan recognises, retroactively, that after 1953 (the aforementioned Seminar I) he comes to occupy the place of a teacher (MT p. 6). Of course, Lacan is referring to his position as a teacher of psychoanalytic method, theory and practice—not something that we are necessarily discussing in this book that is more concerned with education in a broader and more everyday sense. Nevertheless, the centrality of teaching in this talk, alongside numerous references throughout Lacan's oeuvre, makes visible the trace of a more radical position, that of education's irredeemability.

The psychoanalytic discoveries of the unconscious, the death drive, and its fatal wound to enlightenment thinking examined and rethought by Lacan, stand as a great obstacle for educational thought. No wonder, then, perhaps, that psychoanalysis remains repressed in most educational circles. Yet psychoanalysis attends to an essential gap in education, a gap that is not to be filled, but rather accommodated through the mode of psychoanalytical thinking. We thus repeat the words of Austrian psychoanalyst Bruno Bettelheim's essay on teachers and education, himself repeating Freud, 'that psychoanalytic insight be brought to all teachers' (1969, p. 74)—a suggestion that has been almost completely ignored. Bettelheim recognises the impossibility of this call but upholds the utility of psychoanalysis in recognising the traumas and psychic repression of teachers so to allow them to better educate their students. Again, putting teachers on the couch is not our goal—though certainly it may help many in the teaching profession. The teacher (fantasmatically, Symbolically, and historically), might well benefit from psychoanalytic scrutiny.

We do not refute the *position* of teacher, nor seek to depose that minor form of sovereignty here, as is common in more radical educational approaches such as critical pedagogy and child centred learning, even if such a figure is decentred by the Lacanian perspective. Despite the authors' ontological critique of the enterprise of education (Peim & Stock, 2022; Peim, 2012, 2020, 2022; Stock, 2021, 2023), we still address (with a positive interest) the figure or subject of the teacher (though likely for very different reasons from most educationalists). Speaking from our own subjective place as teachers—both in universities and schools, we contend like Shoshana Felman (1982, p. 35) that there is an erotics to teaching, an enjoyment that is to be found in few other places. This erotics is not meant in the quotidian sense of the word, but rather, psychoanalytically speaking, a space in which our drives can be directed, a place of enjoyment that is thrilling and terrifying[2]—corresponding to something Freud sees in the creation of great works of art, for example (SE XXI). It is in passing through this signifier of enjoyment that we are drawn to Lacan, seduced even: he spends much of the latter part of his prolific career teaching analysts about the concept of *jouissance,* a word that loosely translates to enjoyment but with valences of suffering and orgasm. For us, the 'erotical experience' (Felman, 1982, p. 35) of teaching is to be put in a difficult dialogue with the signifier 'education', something we will elucidate as we continue in this book through the concepts of enjoyment/jouissance.

It is likely that most of the readers of this book will have some familiarity with Lacan already, though if not, a glossary of Lacanian terms is appended to support understanding the complexity of his thought. To be brief, Jacques Lacan was a twentieth century psychoanalyst who sought to challenge the field's dominant paradigms of theory and practice. His view, as we see it, was that psychoanalysis had moved too far from the writings of Sigmund Freud and demanded a return to Freud in its movement forward. There is a psychoanalytic structure to this position, as it is only by (re)tracing the past that one can move forward. But Lacan did not merely repeat Freud. Rather, he read Freud in a way that synthesised the philosophy and theory of modernism and modernity, initially through the lens of Ferdinand de Saussure's theory of the signifier and Roman Jakobson's linguistics. What's more, Lacan was steeped in modern philosophy from Descartes to Heidegger. It is perhaps for this reason that Lacan is often upheld in philosophy circles as a significant contributor to 'post-structuralism' alongside Derrida and Foucault, the context where both authors of this book first encountered Lacan (even if we do not fully condone this generic division). He produced only one book, the notoriously impenetrable *Écrits,* mostly delivering his theories through seminars for twenty-eight years of new material. As will be made clear in this chapter and beyond, Lacan saw himself (albeit unconventionally) as a teacher more than a writer.

Return to Freud

Just as it was Lacan's endeavour to return to Freud, we will occasionally do so ourselves. It is no surprise that Freud, like Lacan, takes aim at education (Britzman, 1991, 2009, 2015; Taubman, 2012; Lapping, 2020). In

[2] See also Amia Srinivasan's *The Right to Sex* (2021) which also examines the complexity of pedagogy and Eros, partly though psychoanalytic ideas.

Freud, we already find the kernel of educational critique that took force in the radical educational movements of the twentieth century such as deschooling and critical pedagogy. Arguably, there is a radicality to Freud's analysis of education that remains unheard, particularly concerning his discovery of the death drive.

Freud's late work, *Civilization and its Discontents*, bristles with barbs about the state of social institutions in their relation to pleasure. The broad thesis of the essay is that the formation of civilization necessarily entails the trading of untethered pleasure for safety, security and sociality. But in this exchange, some pleasure must remain. A 'mild narcosis' (SE XXI, p. 81) must be offered by social institutions, the process of education being one of them. Previously, in Freud's 1909 lectures at Clark University, he had stated 'the whole trend of your previous education and all your habits of thought are inevitably bound to make you into opponents of psychoanalysis, and how much you would have to overcome in yourselves in order to get the better of this instinctive opposition' (SE XV, I). Freud takes aim here not just at schools as was to be done in the next half of the twentieth by the thinkers of liberatory forms of pedagogy, but also at education in the big sense, a perhaps previously unthinkable idea. Freud makes clear that education in modernity is a process of taming untethered pleasure and closing an attunement to the unconscious—two things that may be intertwined.

But it is in Freud's lesser-read essay 'Wild Psycho-analysis' that the most radical ('anarchistic' says Malabou (2023)) perspectives on education arise. It is worth recounting at length here, as we find it inflicts a devastating wound on education that educationists still seek to repress. The essay begins with Freud recalling a patient who had recently divorced her husband and considering her interaction with another analyst, one who mistook 'sexual life … [as] the need for coitus or analogous acts producing orgasm and emission of the sexual substances' (SE XI, p. 222). The previous analyst suggested that the patient might find a new husband or masturbate to 'cure' her anxiety. Freud's concern in this case is that the analyst in question neglected the patient's sublimation of desire, where the 'concept of what is sexual comprises far more; it goes lower and also higher than its popular sense' (p. 222). Indeed, 'satisfactions … can often find only very inadequate outlet in coitus and other sexual acts' (p. 223). Freud thus posits that the analyst 'over-estimate[s] his influence' (p. 224) on the patient. He does not engage in psychoanalysis, as such, but rather offers to pass on his wisdom to teach her how to get better. Herein lies the educational corollary. The analyst attempts to know the 'signs' (p. 224) of the patient's hysteria so to offer a 'remedy' (p. 225), rather than focussing on and exploring the form it takes. Thus:

> It is a long superseded idea, and one derived from superficial appearances, that the patient suffers from a sort of ignorance, and that if one removes this ignorance by giving him information … he is bound to recover. The pathological factor is not his ignorance in *itself*, but the root of this ignorance in his *inner resistances*; it was they that first called this ignorance into being, and they still maintain it now. The task of the treatment lies in combating these resistances. Informing the patient of what he does not *know* because he has repressed it is only one of the necessary preliminaries to the treatment. If knowledge about the unconscious were as important for the patient as people inexperienced in psychoanalysis imagine, listening to lectures or reading books would be enough to cure him. (p. 225)

Analysis is here described not as a path from ignorance to knowledge (the very same Symbolic logic found in almost all imaginaries of education), but rather a constant reinvestigation of psychic resistances. Traversing unconscious material, as opposed to reading books and attending lectures, is the way of psychoanalysis. Perhaps, we might even venture to say that the sort of pursuit of knowledge Freud criticizes here fosters a monastic servility to the book (Peim, 2022)—the formation of the helpless 'civilized' subject. We may even go further to say that this pursuit of knowledge from ignorance may intensify psychic disorders, as does the 'wild psychoanalysis' that Freud equates with education.

Ultimately, a Lacanian teacher, like Freud in his consideration of 'wild psychoanalysis', must engage with education as a thing that will arouse questions concerning fantasy, imaginaries, desires, symbols, and trauma, and, most pressingly, with 'the thing itself'. To understand what we mean, let us return briefly to Lacan's recognition of his teaching and the way he situates himself in this subject position:

> In the beginning, there was not the origin. There was the place … Place … in the sense of structure … the place I have come to, which puts me in a position to teach. (MT, pp. 4–5)

What Lacan raises here is that the 'source' of becoming a teacher is of little interest. Indeed, 'one always talks rubbish when it comes to origins' (MT, p. 33), that is, there is no inciting incident or singular moment that one decides, consciously or unconsciously, to become a teacher, even if trainees are regularly required to write statements about 'what made you want to become a teacher?' No, teaching is a retroactive subject position for Lacan, made in looking back, formed from and by the place or space that one occupies. Simply by being put in in a position to teach (whatever that might mean), one is able to be a teacher. Any account of teaching is therefore inextricably bound to that sense of place wherein teachers reside. For us, this raises the essential background to an understanding of our position on the Lacanian teacher through an approach to the (too-often ignored) ontology of education.

Lacan's Ontology

We here draw heavily on the philosophical strings to Lacan's bow, though Lacan can be read in relation to many other disciplines too (biology, maths, anthropology, and so on). This is not simply because we are interested in philosophy as authors, but rather because of the philosophical dimension of education that stretches back to Ancient Greece and beyond. The very possibility of what we might call education is of ontological concern (what *is* education?), and indeed the philosopher is often, says a string of pessimists from Diogenes to Cioran, compelled to teach their philosophy to others. Those that challenge this compulsion offer a 'rival mode of existence that runs counter to the beneficent humanism of liberal education' (Allen, 2020, p. 43), appear to us 'a phenomenon alien to this earth' (Cioran, 2018, p. 5). Philosophy of education, philosophy as education, education of philosophy, all pertain to a particular selection of the philosophical canon and a way of reading it that both pessimism and Lacan challenge—as will we with our educational thoughts. This begins with a consideration of ontology.

Lacanian ontology is very much a product of what we might loosely refer to as an ontological turn in philosophy through Heidegger and Freud, especially, although also informed by the philosophical tradition though Descartes, Spinoza, Kant and Hegel. Some thinkers in the psychoanalytic tradition are reluctant to use the term ontology—a term subject to much conflict and misuse. Heidegger—a figure of such interest to Lacan he was invited to stay with him—proposes the way we understand it: as the philosophy of Being. Zupančič interestingly relates the phenomenological with the ontological when she asserts that the question of 'Why does something appear as it appears?' (Zupančič & Terada, 2015, p. 15) is at once ontological and Lacanian. 'I am what I is' (XVI, p. 55) says Lacan at one point: implying perhaps that the subject is always already a subject of Being. Lacan's use of the term, like many others, is variable throughout his career. In one formulation ontology is highlighted, perhaps ironically, as the 'use of the copula' (XX, p. 31), a connecting word between subject and complement: 'be' being the paradigm case.

Our work in the past has been almost solely dedicated to ontological questions concerning education that we continue here through Lacan:

> 'How does education stand with being?'
> 'How does education *be*?'

The ontological question concerning education, the question of what education is in our world and in our time is almost entirely foreclosed, even, if not especially, in the philosophy of education. A main aim of this book is to rethink conventional understandings of what education is and can be through what we might refer to provisionally as a Lacanian ontology, a 'way of thinking' that we believe can address the most intimate experience of being in education as well as the most comprehensive understanding of the global phenomenon of education. A Lacanian teacher as we outline it situates themself *in* this ontology, but cannot be outside of it.

Lacan's rethinking of Freud, then, is informed by currents in Kant, Hegel and Heidegger, among others, where questions concerning subjectivity are extensively and rigorously addressed. The legacy of enlightenment, through the densely elaborated thinking of Kant, had generated a split between knowledge and existence and, in effect, between subject and object. Kant had concluded in *The Critique of Pure Reason* that an ineradicable distinction must pertain between what we know as subjects and what exists independently of our perception ('phenonemenon' and 'noumenon'). This epistemological difference haunts western metaphysics with an enduring force that continues to trouble all those modes of thinking that lay claim to a certain grip on reality, that affirm that the foundations of knowledge can be absolute, secure and incontrovertible, independent of any subjective dimension (Meillasoux, 2009).

We'll see later how Lacanian thinking has a bearing on the paradigm form of knowledge for our time, science, as a mode of knowing in relation to being. Kant's intricate phenomenology had determined that our knowledge must partake of an element of appearance that precludes any claim to an immediate or acquired grasp of the essential substance of whatever it is that takes our interest or concern. For Kant we must concede that we may grasp phenomena (things-as-they-appear) but that noumena (things-in-themselves) elude our certain grasp even while we apprehend their certain existence. While part of the 'problem' lies in the logic of subject and object (and world) relations, another dimension puts into question our own identification with ourselves as simply thinking, ratiocinative selves. Before Kant, Descartes had found the one certainty that might found some sure basis for knowledge in the cogito: 'I think therefore I am'. This thinking subject is still the dominant way we picture teachers and students in the processes of education, one that can be coherently traced and thus mastered through some form of pedagogy.

Still, while Cartesian/Kantian consciousness of the subject might be the condition for my perceptions, beliefs and ability to navigate my way through my world as a knowing being, consciousness can also be conceived of as a sort of confinement, an enclosure that limits my apprehension of things isolating me from other ways of knowing than my own. And how could we determine that the world as it appears to consciousness corresponds to how the world actually is? Only through consciousness. The microscope, like the telescope, revealed things to perception that had been hitherto unknown, disclosing unseen aspects of the world. The implication of this, to put it too tersely, is that our apprehension of things, constrained by consciousness, cannot be taken on trust as how things are. This seems to be bad news for the aspirations of both epistemology and ontology to have a certain grasp of the nature of things. From the very start of his career (I, p. 225), Lacan unsettled the ontological narrative of the telescope that seemed to claim things could be carefully observed and ordered through processes of reasoning. As his thinking developed in his teaching, we see the complexifying of an onto-topology[3] in his three registers of Imaginary, Symbolic and Real—dimensions that retain the tensions inherent in phenomenology, ontology and epistemology in all their intricate and dynamic relations and offer something more than the philosophers Lacan was indebted to.

The aporetic condition of both knowing and being that are implicit through Lacan's thinking—with its emphasis on the 'promethean' (E, p. 201) unconscious and the dislocated orders of being—amplifies the

[3] Here we refer to both the ontological—referring to Being, and the topological—referring to three-dimensional space. Lacan regularly uses topology to redescribe his RSI ontology, such as in the Möbius strip, the Klein bottle, or the Borromean knot. In these spaces, one is never on top or below, inside or out, just as with the subject of RSI.

various blows to the project of enlightenment and its handmaiden, rationality, problematizing in turn the enlightenment legacy and its subject, 'humanity'. Following Kant, Hegel had struggled to salvage the enlightenment desire for universal knowledge, proclaiming a faith that history unfolded progressively, even while acknowledging that his historicism implied cultural relativism. Hegel's highly abstract solution was to abstract the proper object of knowledge from the world to consciousness of the world. 'Reason is the certainty of consciousness that it is all reality' so that the great task is for rational consciousness to fully know itself (Belsey, 2004, p. 23). On this view the destiny of reason was to hold reality together and render truth conscious of itself as its own world and of the world as itself. This theological celebration of Geist, that remains audible in some educational discourses, got problematized through various strands of thinking that Lacan inherited, including Freud's intense and abiding skepticism and Heidegger's critique of ontotheology. The project of enlightenment rationality that prevails in education's more salvific and redemptive moments, likewise seems to be radically at odds with Lacan's engagement with fundamental ontology that gets construed through an original rethinking of the relations between language and being.

The Three Registers

The originality of Lacanian ontology enables a dynamic rethinking of the most fundamental relations between subjects, objects, worlds, World, language, ideas and being. The intricacies of the relations between those various dimensions of 'being' are held in a mobile and dynamic tension in the articulation of three orders, orders that co-exist, overlap and interfere with one another constantly. Lacan's reformulation of what Heidegger referred to as the question of questions, the '*Seinsfrage*' (2008), the most primordial and persistent of questions, is not performed systematically but emerges in and from the *Écrits* and the seminars. It takes shape as a kind of three-dimensional mapping of ontological space, that is the space of the subject's being, but also the space of any object's being and the being of being, or world. Lacanian ontology, then, enables an approach to any object of inquiry—such as the classroom, the school, teaching, the teacher, the curriculum, knowledge—to be situated within a topography that articulates the interactions it will be enframed by in the Real, Symbolic, and Imaginary (RSI).[4]

[4] Lacan does not capitalise each register, though as many do, we choose to here to prevent confusion with more everyday uses of the words.

The reverberations of Heidegger's fundamental ontology echo through Lacan's implicit ontology and in his various formulations of the relations between the Real the Symbolic and the Imaginary, although in many ways Lacan's RSI has a sophistication that cuts out some of the more questionable elements in Heidegger, such as the affirmation of authenticity. But Lacan's barred subject that we examine later is not too distant a relation to Heidegger's *dasein*, a subject who is radically contingent or 'thrown', beset by anxiety, absorbed in care for the contingently ordered world of its dwelling that constitutes a horizon for its conscious grasp of things.

None of the dimensions of RSI is reducible to the other. They coexist at the level of the subject's encounter with the object in the context of their specific world, defined within given co-ordinates of time, place and form. The most mundane encounters, events, experiences can be understood in terms of the threefold torsion of these orders of Being.

> elementary registers, whose foundations I have since laid, known as the symbolic, the imaginary, and the real… (E, p. 310)

At the Imaginary level we identify ourselves and the things, events ideas we encounter through unconscious projections, reading our world and ourselves within a powerfully emotionally-laden, usually tacit understanding. Our apprehension of 'things'—including very big entities such as 'the very nature of things'—is necessarily caught up with this Imaginary order, a mode of relation that can't be erased by, for example, a rationalist or scientific stance. A cliched scientist gazing down a microscope to look at minute cells in a living organism also has an Imaginary relation with the object she observes and perhaps pursues, as well as the relation determined by the historically shifting Symbolic order of biological sciences that more formally and explicitly perhaps shapes her encounter with those objects. The scientist's world determines the procedures, the categories for thinking (the discourse) that will animate her microscopic examination but there is something else at work, above and beyond the purely scientific discourse. This other, crucial, dimension—the dimension of desire—operates at the level of how the scientist perceives herself as a scientist and at the level of whatever status she may hold within her specific world within the larger world of science within *the* World at large.

One aspect of this might be understood as the Imaginary mastery of the object that the practice she engages with offers, that the scientific discourse enables, that may afford a sense of purpose to her role within an institution, and a world (possibly at several levels). We could expand our speculations on the Imaginary identifications at work in this scenario: perhaps she sees herself, consciously or otherwise, as engaged in an important project dedicated to the improvement of an aspect of life, perhaps also sensing her work to be in a tradition of worthy scientific endeavour, forging a pathway of knowledge in the grander, big project of human progress? Fantasies are clearly littered throughout the Imaginary, including the narratives we keep telling ourselves personally, or publicly in cinema and television. A story of progress like this is not hard to find in the Imaginary of education, too, another Imaginary pathway of human progress towards better things in the endlessly deferred future. The Imaginary, in Lacan's implicit ontology, at several levels including both the fundamental and the grand level, holds the world of the scientist (and the educationist) together.[5]

The Symbolic order, inherited through language in general, with its institutionalized semantic categories and regulated by grammatical combinations, appears in more specific ways through discourses that 'form the objects of which they speak', giving weight to the collective order, conceived not as a monolithically controlling force, but rather as both an enclosure of and a clearing for the possibilities for thinking, knowing and being. The Symbolic order is historically, culturally and even locally shifting as well as conflicted, yet it carries with it a constraining power that exerts a significant element of sovereignty over thinking, both conscious and unconscious. As Lacan says, the Symbolic is 'the major determination the subject receives from the itinerary of a signifier' (E, p. 7). We should also note that the Symbolic is akin to what Lacan calls *Autre*, Other with a capital O and thus known as 'the big Other' in translation. This term reframes the Symbolic as an entity that, though does not exist, feels like an entity of radical otherness, difference, that can thus verify what we say and do. When we speak, we must pass through the Symbolic, the treasure

[5] Louis Althusser's formulation of ideological state apparatuses (1971) and their relations with intimate aspects of the self, took enough from both Freud and Lacan to offer a serious rethinking of some fundamental Marxist ideas, in an attempt to revivify Marxist thought with a new, contemporary philosophical depth. Althusser's account of the interpellation of the subject, as an explanation of social identity and being, owes a powerful debt to Lacanian phenomenology reset into wider historical, social conditions. Althusser had attended Lacan's seminars.

trove of signifiers, and thus 'the locus of the Other, the Other as witness' (E, p. 684). We must be able to imagine a being that has every signifier that we might use, and hence when we use them, we do so under the gaze of that being.

The dominant assumptions that prevail about education can be seen as a manifestation of the Symbolic order: assumptions about education's benignity, about its essential contribution to social order, well-being and flourishing. There are powerfully embedded assumptions in the Symbolic order about education as good for the individual, as necessary for a full and purposeful life, as well as being essential to producing law-abiding and self-governing subjects within any given polity. In addition, there are the claims made, usually by educationists, that only education can save the world, can generate fulfilment and can ensure progress, improvement, enlightenment and so on. This varied set of positive beliefs is not set out in any handbook for thinking, but is well established in the everyday discourses of educational ideas and ideology and, in many cases, of educational practice too. There are of course exceptions to this: the positive image of education is not shared by all. The Symbolic order must also be the grounds for a contest of ideas, even while certain ideas dominate. At the level of language, the world is always already ordered according to syntax and grammar that set the categories and the modes of their arrangement, although this order may be historically and culturally shifted. At the level of discourse, an array of forces come into play to both stabilize meaning and to allow for a degree of mobility and invention.

The teacher in the classroom is beset by a certain powerful and powerfully constraining Symbolic order. There is, for examples, age stratification, the configuration of space, the staged ordering of the day into discrete lessons, the curriculum, with its stages, specifications for knowledge and pedagogy, and the requirement for lesson planning, the expectation of a disciplinary order. All these features have to be negotiated by the individual teacher. Within the stable ordering of time, place and conduct the teacher must negotiate their own mode of being, always under various external pressures from the managerial, administrative and disciplinary regimes that intersect. There is a multi-faceted discourse, including a pedagogic discourse partly concerned with the delivery of the curriculum, partly also concerned with the mode of being of the teacher, a discourse that constitutes worlds of objects and modes of relating to them. What we might call the technology of pedagogy must be addressed (as we will do in Chap. 4), including dealing with the physical paraphernalia—the arrangement of desks, the distribution of teaching materials, the competent deployment of display systems. Much of this becomes, with 'hard use' the ingrained world of the teacher, attuned to the environment and its intense Symbolic configuration.

Spatially the school, while often rendered shabby by overuse and cheap construction, is highly ordered. The essential Symbolic spaces can be traced to the emergence of the elementary nineteenth century school, although school topography has become transformed, refined and subtilized. The quintessential architecture of the classic 'board' school, often constructed in grand style, was constructed around its key elements: playground, hall and classroom (Peim, 2001). Even while the 'real' spatial arrangement might differ, these retain their governmental and Symbolic functions (Stock, 2024). As Lacan declares in *Écrits*:

> what distinguishes the architecture from the building: namely, a logical power that governs [*ordonne*] the architecture beyond what the building allows for by way of possible utilization. Thus no building, unless reduced to the merest of barracks, can do without this order that makes it akin to discourse. (E, p. 586)

Lacanian ontology, we might say, however, does not determine such architecture (emphasizing the *arche*) monolithic and deterministic. Architecture can be and often is, of course, reinscribed, refunctioned in relation to shifts in the Symbolic order, and shifts, we might add in the Imaginary register that provides an element of collective desire to the order that pertains.

The classroom, interestingly organized much like the space of a theatre (as we will assert regularly in this book) inherits Symbolic and Imaginary properties from its architectural arrangement. This was clear with the dais in early classrooms, an actual platform of the teacher. But now, in the late twentieth century after the dais has mostly disappeared, the imposition of performance and audience can be subtly adapted to shifting Symbolic world of education that it sits within. The impulse to perform onstage and seek the Imaginary identification with the material being taught in the lesson remains at play (Stock, 2024). The playground even more vividly illustrates this dimension of the relations between architecture and function, even where 'playground' no longer necessarily designates a certain demarcated space. The playground has been described (Hunter, 1994) as the morally managed space where the culture of the school meets with and seeks to modify the culture of the child. Another way to look at it would be in the meeting of modes of the Symbolic orders inflected by the various forms of the Imaginary at work. Children play games, adults supervise and seek to modify behaviour at the level of disposition. We might transpose this simple account into more complex scenes where institutions offer 'free' recreational spaces with the intention of affording opportunities for the relaxed modification not just of conduct but also of habit and inclination.[6]

In Lacanian ontology, though, an exhaustive account of the elements of the social space of the educational setting would not be enough to furnish a full description of the mode of being of the teacher in context. Negotiating the timetable, the curriculum, the display regime, pedagogical relations, social relations—all engage with the psychic apparatus that animates the subject. Manifestations of the Imaginary reverberate in all aspects of the teacher's being. This is experienced intensely by the initiate teacher who is scrutinized, frequently under observation to test not just specific competences in managing classroom relations and in delivering the curriculum but also to scrutinize the demeanour of the delivery, the pacing of pedagogic time, the savoir-faire of the discourse. In the formation of the teacher observation is explicit. Identity is at stake, the initiate teacher must engage in reflexive self-analysis to demonstrate the learning process at work in becoming that special form of self, the teacher proper. A telling moment in the film *Dangerous Minds* occurs when LouAnne Johnson, the hero teacher, struggling with a difficult class of 'reluctant learners' sits at home reading a famous teaching manual, throws it aside, dons her leather jacket and poses in front of the mirror as though testing out this new role, her new identity to see herself, as it were, as a teacher, but not as a teacher defined by the handbook, rather as a leather-jacket-wearing teacher attuned to the needs and the life-worlds of her charges.

Being seen, and seeing oneself, are fundamental elements of the Lacanian ontology that not only address a conventional phenomenology of self and other but that also include the element of the 'gaze': a crucial component that belongs mostly to the Imaginary dimension in Lacanian

[6] In classic descriptions of good pedagogy, Vygotsky's 'zone of proximal development', peddled in teacher training the world over, is analogous to the playground space as the psychic region wherein new knowledge can only inhere by engaging with existing knowledge. In Lacanian terms we might subtilize this account by making reference to the modification, extension and refinement of the Symbolic order in a process that also seeks to engage the Imaginary via a desire that is activated in positive, developmental terms.

ontology. Once again, the architecture of the classroom engenders the gaze via its arrangement as a theatrical space always already seen by an audience (be that the teacher or the student), a mirror, an 'exchange of gazes' (E, p. 55). At the level of the Imaginary the teacher sees and is constantly seen, configured in the world of the institution that is not only out there as a specific and actual place and space but that is configured in being seen as a certain kind of space with a certain tenor, inscribed with meaning, feeling and the complex projections of the subject. There is no cool, detached, purely analytic stance for the subject in this relation: 'the gaze is clearly the object that presents each desire with its universal rule, by materializing its cause, in binding to it the subject's division "between center and absence"' (E, pp. 662–663), that is, what is seen is always populated, as it were, with this psychic material. And, of course, teachers will often describe the feeling they have on approaching or on entering a building that has been the place of their work, where work includes this element of accommodating to the emotional and identity laden charge that the particular context holds for the subject. One may approach the school where one teaches, where one is a teacher, with complex and varied sensations, laden with memories, images, that are viscerally experienced, held between conscious and unconscious apprehension. An incident that occurred yesterday, a difficult class last year, a troubling conversation with a colleague last week: what one sees as one approaches cannot be reduced to a decisively adumbrated visual image. The 'act' of seeing is fraught with meaning that is the effect of the relations between object and subject. This is the effect of the gaze: our subject being is caught up in the field of vision.

But the Imaginary does not only operate at the visceral level of involuntary feeling. As LouAnne Johnson looks at herself in her fetching leather jacket in the mirror, at home, she is trying on the mantle of a teacher type through the 'bric-a-brac' (III, p. 155) of the Imaginary. She is engaging in a common fantasy that lends possible meaning to the role she is struggling to accommodate herself to and chime with. We might speculate that she is also trying to fit herself into a role that engages with education as a field of potential salvation, as she seeks to offer something to her charges above and beyond the relatively deprived lives of the social context they inhabit. She will need to become creative, inventive, agile and canny: so she projects this possible self to herself in the name of conducting or at least contributing to this mission. The Imaginary is at work, animating LouAnne Johnson's initiation (in a similar tension found in Ryan Gosling's crack pipe in *Half Nelson,* a film examined in Chap. 3) into the world of education, via the specific portal of the 'academy' class of the 'public' school she is now employed at. So we can see the Imaginary operating at several levels here: as a basic fantasy concerning what I might want to be, but also in a bigger sense, having far-reaching effects in the Real, as a fantasmatic idea of what I am a part of as I adapt my being to the being of the teacher I want to become, feeding my impulsion and giving it some specific shape. The jacket metonymically comes to indicate becoming, not just any old cog-in-the-wheel, brick-in-the-wall teacher, but the cool, accessible teacher attuned to the world and the perspective of her students all the better not merely to teach them some'thing', some element of the curriculum, but to help them learn to be their better selves in a transformational process.

Imaginary identification occurs classically through the ego, but doesn't have to be constantly explicitly conscious to be effective. We might add that the ego itself is significantly composed of such identifications, including Imaginary identification we make with an ideal version of ourselves. In *Écrits* (p. 265), Lacan refers to the 'Imaginary matrix' as a kind of generative and persistent 'moment' that engages the subject in the process of engaging with the Symbolic order, through the Imaginary order. LouAnne Johnson's moment of half-conscious realization in *Dangerous Minds* where she dons the jacket and realizes that maybe she can, in a meaningful way, give herself to the business of being a teacher does not accidentally involve a mirror. The specular image is important for Lacan's explication of Imaginary identifications as it creates the visual illusion of a certain wholeness that comes, even if momentarily, and thereafter sporadically, to represent the wholeness of the subject to herself. So there may be a frisson of pleasure, a feeling of satisfaction in self-realization that while founded in an illusion, and therefore alienating, accords with significant elements in the Symbolic order. The subject is enraptured by its own image as belonging to what is above and beyond itself. Imaginary identifications are not arbitrary. They partake of the Symbolic order and are strongly enmeshed in language belonging to the realm of the signified, caught up in signification's mobilization of the signifier/signified relation. Language has both Symbolic and Imaginary aspects, so that meaning is always laden with Imaginary identification and projection and language has that captivating power. The mode of speech of the teacher with its special inflections, its assumption of authority, its interrogative modes and its directive statements is evidence of the capture of the teacher by the discourse of the

Other, including that frisson of enjoyment in attaining to something of the Imaginary model.

In short, we find the Symbolic and Imaginary vividly at work in the day-to-day of education, where some subjects identify and are identified as 'students' with others as 'teachers' in 'learning spaces' like 'classrooms' where 'progress' happens via 'pedagogy' and is punctuated by 'assessment', and so on. There is a grammatical pattern, as it were, to the shape and ordering of the signifiers that constitute the Symbolic order of education, but like in the syntax of grammar, there is also a direction. This direction is that of an upward curve towards something—a punctuating signifier such as 'progress', 'future', 'career', or even simply 'being educated', all galvanized by the Imaginary, with some sometimes failing, and falling, out of the circle. Students are regularly told that 'even if this is boring and irrelevant, it makes you a more rounded human being!' Thus, the claim goes in the classroom, that if the signifiers above interact as 'they should', the subjects of education will go on to prosperity and happiness (and so might we all).

Into the Real

Perhaps the most elusive and the most intriguing of Lacan's three orders of being is the Real: as 'that which subsists outside of symbolization' (E, p. 324).

> the real does not wait [attend], especially not for the subject, since it expects [attend] nothing from speech. But it is there, identical to his existence, a noise in which one can hear anything and everything, ready to submerge with its roar what the 'reality principle' constructs there that goes by the name of the 'outside world.' (p. 324)

The Real is difficult to define perhaps except in terms of the brute reality of 'stuff' that lies beyond the order of symbolization, as the undifferentiated material of being. Of course, it is ever present: it is the ground of our being without us being able to access it directly. The transforming, differentiating, ordering effects of 'the signifier' indicate, beyond themselves, the brute reality of our being in the Real. Animated, driven by the Imaginary and Symbolic, we bump up against the Real in its intransigent materiality, in its mindless and implacable exertion of forces and materials beyond our control or ken.

> For the real, whatever upheaval we subject it to, is always and in every case in its place; it carries its place stuck to the sole of its shoe, there being nothing that can exile it from it. (E, p. 22)

It is the encounter with this thing stuck to the sole of the shoe that is most horrifying to educationists, indicating that something else lurks amidst the neatly ordered arrangement of educational logics, pedagogies, architectures, curricula, and so on, something else that escapes understanding or control. Indeed, encounters with the Real are likely to be fraught with fear, beset by loss of meaning. In the absence of the Symbolic a kind of primordial materiality takes precedence. To borrow from Derrida (2001), we may experience the Real also as a kind of present absence, as in the case of the death of another, or as an absent presence, someone physically there but inaccessible to us. One author's father, still a powerful figure in the Symbolic order, no longer exists in the category of the Real, though a trace of him remains Real in the unconscious. This example enforces some recognition of the relation between symbolization and death. The Symbolic order obscures, as it were, by shifting the being of the thing to the signifier, at the same time as granting it a place in the formal order of things, articulated through linguistic difference. As Lacan insists, the Real is indifferent to the Symbolic order. It persists in being shapeless, formless but palpably there and usually uncanny when encountered. What's more the Real is to be distinguished from 'reality' (the world picture that culture presents to us) being primordial, totally divorced from and inaccessible to the Symbolic. We can speculate on the contours of reality but the Real is beyond our adumbrations appearing only as an incomprehensible intrusion into the world as we know it and expect it to be.[7]

The final scenes of the 2011 film *Detachment* depict a substitute teacher played by Adrian Brody reading aloud to his class. He first describes the 'weight' that he feels when he walks through the corridors of the school—the intrusion of the Real into the neatness of the Symbolic order of education. He reads an extract from Poe's *The Fall of the House of Usher* that

[7] The world as we experience it, our world, the world of the classroom say or the school or the university, as well as *the* world is thrown into relief by language as a more or less ordered structure of things that makes entities visible as different, if related. In language for Heidegger, as with the Sapir-Whorf hypothesis, language corresponds with the world of 'a people' in their historical constitution. And while language positively clarifies and brings the sayable into being, it also, thereby, generates the unsayable, the dark shadow of the visible, as it were, that lies beyond (Heidegger, 1971, p. 74).

describes the decay and rot of the estate, and the 'iciness, a sinking, a sickening of the heart' that pervades the scene. As Brody reads, the scene cuts to a montage of the school in the same state of rot and decay: overturned chairs, dark classrooms, reports and exam papers whirling around the hallways. It would be easy to see this as simply a lament at the loss of 'proper education' in American schools, but we can see it differently as the educational Real that always refuses our acknowledgment, a swirling void of disorganized stuff that is endlessly tamed through the Symbolic and Imaginary dimensions teachers uphold.

We might also consider the unthinkable vastness of the cosmos, unknowable in its immensity, or, alternatively, we might consider the inscrutable, perhaps unnerving look of the animal that we can only make sense of in our (non-animal) terms (Derrida, 2008). As what lies beyond culture, language, the Real is there (ever-present) but remains unknowable, enigmatic, disturbing. It needn't be quite so abstract as illustrated above: for the teacher, the 'real' teacher, not LouAnne Johnson in *Dangerous Minds* or Mr. Keating in *Dead Poets Society*, manifestations of the Real may appear in quite familiar form when the educational Symbolic order fails to hold up and when the Imaginary fantasy flags or fails: when the mundane brute disorder of the school environment shows itself in the obscene figure illicitly drawn on the whiteboard, or when the insouciant pupil mimics the teacher behind her back, when the litter-obsessed deputy-head bawls out a wanton pupil for their sheer absence of care and investment in the proper order of things. All teachers could testify to such moments, events or phenomena that betray the intrusion of the Real into the fantasmatically scaffolded Symbolic order and the feeling of deflation that attends. These lesions in the Symbolic order indicate a breakdown of the alliance between fantasy and symbolization; in the absence of these animating elements, sense of purpose can drain away, all seems flat and meaningless. There is a constant effort, though, to reduce the intrusions of the Real, to keep the Real at bay as it were. At a school one of us visited as teacher training tutor, pupils sought to undermine the explicit domination of the school Symbolic order by wearing their compulsory uniform neckties with a cut that rendered them both compliant and subversive. The school had commissioned a deputy head to harangue pupils who wore their neckties at half-mast, so the pupils, mostly neatly uniformed and obedient, used the cut tie to express some break in the governmental regime.

Navigating the School

Cracks appear in the Symbolic, then, and it is in these cracks that we glimpse the Real. The school fire drill perhaps best exemplifies the ordering of the Symbolic order and something of its automaton-like characteristic, rather like the everyday operations of the timetable involving the self-guided movement of pupils through an often-intricate topography. In a well-ordered school environment, the fire-drill manages itself. Pupils *en masse* gather into their age-stratified groupings to submit themselves for a registration that itself confirms bureaucratically that they are securely where they ought to be. It is the same registration system, often now electronic, that charts their progress, differentiates them into their 'proper' categories and carries the indelible account of their progress through attainment targets of the taxonomized knowledge embodied in the centrally defined curriculum. Ideally, things are in their places, the proper prevails and the educational Symbolic order grinds out its classificatory schema.

Of course, the Symbolic order is not (quite) totalitarian. The maverick teacher knows how to navigate both the disciplinary order and the constraints of the curriculum. The classroom, for all its enclosed cellular character, can offer a space for movement and to some degree for being otherwise. There is always something that resists symbolization. The canny teacher understands this just as does the recalcitrant pupil. The Imaginary may identify differently, shifting the focus of the Symbolic order, creating its own terminology and taxonomy, as Paul Willis's classic ethnography of 'lads' in a West Midlands school attests (1977) and as what is at stake in Bernstein's distinctions in 'code theory' (1975) or in Bourdieu's account of 'habitus' (1977). The psychoanalytic account of the orders or registers of being in Lacan correspond powerfully with these perspectives and offer extensions and refinements to their grasp of the dynamics of educational social relations.

Educational institutions are fraught with a fear of indiscipline and any breakdown of the Symbolic order may be experienced as a threat to the integrity of the enterprise. University teachers bemoan falling standards of various kinds, qualification inflation, and the cultural impoverishment of their charges. In schools the worst nightmare for the individual teacher and the institution is loss of discipline. In both contexts challenges to authority must be contested and the order of things maintained, an order that is enacted contextually, symbolically, every day in all the little and big rituals that pertain to these worlds of education that subsist on their repetition: taking the register, morning assembly, the end-of-lesson and beginning of lesson rituals, the choreography of movement through the day. But there are grander rituals too that Symbolically hold educational worlds together ensuring the Symbolic order is renewed and refreshed. In the university perhaps the most value-laden ritual is the PhD viva in which not only is the quality of the thesis subject to peer critique and review, but the person of the candidate is also put under question. At stake is the very integrity of the knowledge production function of the institution, invested with powerfully Imaginary proprieties. The candidate must submit to the Symbolic order of the ritual and carefully navigate both the presentation of their offering and the conduct of their interrogation. It is difficult to overestimate the significance of this doctoral induction ritual within the Symbolic order of the university. And difficult, too, to overestimate the delicate negotiation required on the part of the inductee to navigate the balance between being required to stand in the place, as it were, of the one-who-knows, and knows authoritatively, and to also accede to the already established authority of the examiners who occupy that Imaginary position in Symbolically clinched form. Meanwhile the Real that is the supposed 'object' of the knowledge procession embodied in the scenario of the viva voce rests implacably, impervious to the impulsions of its participants and all its subjects deigning to respond now and then to the probings of aspiring archons (that we discuss in Chap. 4).

The Lacanian way of thinking, as we've briefly described it here in relation to some key aspects of the world of education, offers a serious and productive disturbance to the given order of things, that is to the Symbolic order of education and of formal educational discourses such as those found in academic contexts, but also to those that inform both policy and ideology. At the same time, a Lacanian perspective offers insight to the various Imaginary identifications that feed the fantasies that sustain the Symbolic order, animating it with desire. Lacanian ideas have a great deal to offer, we believe, in rethinking both education and what it means to be a subject of education, and that subject of education that is the teacher. The existential experience of being a teacher, including the experience of meaning, and loss of meaning, but especially of enjoyment, seem to be especially susceptible to being rethought through the Lacanian perspective.

References

Others

Allen, A. (2020). *Cynicism*. MIT Press.
Althusser, L. (1971). Ideology and Ideological State Apparatuses. In L. Althusser (Ed.), *Lenin and Philosophy and Other Essays*. Monthly Review Press.
Belsey, C. (2004). *Culture and the Real: Theorizing Cultural Criticism* (1st ed.). Routledge.
Bernstein, B. (1975). *Class, Codes and Control: Towards a Theory of Educational Transmission, Volume 3*. Routledge.
Bettelheim, B. (1969). Psychoanalysis and Education. *The School Review, 77*(2), 73–86.
Bourdieu, P. (1977). *Outline of a Theory of Practice*. Cambridge University Press.
Britzman, D. (1991). *Practice Makes Practice: A Critical Study of Learning to Teach*. SUNY Press.
Britzman, D. (2009). *The Very Thought of Education: Psychoanalysis and the Impossible Professions*. SUNY Press.
Britzman, D. (2015). *A Psychoanalyst in the Classroom*. SUNY Press.
Cioran, E.M. (2018 [1975]). *A Short History of Decay*. Penguin Books.
Derrida, J. (2001). *The Work of Mourning*. University of Chicago Press.
Derrida, J. (2008). *The Animal That Therefore I Am* (M.-L. Mallet, Ed.). Fordham University Press.
Ellsworth, E. (1997). *Teaching Positions. Difference, Pedagogy, and the Power of Address*. Teachers College Press.
Felman, S. (1982). Psychoanalysis and Education: Teaching Terminable and Interminable. *Yale French Studies, 63*, 21–44.
Heidegger, M. (1971). *Poetry, Language, Thought* (A. Hofstadter, Trans.). Harper & Rowe.
Heidegger, M. (2008 [1927]). *Being and Time*. HarperCollins.
Hunter, I. (1994). *Rethinking the School: Subjectivity, Bureaucracy, Criticism* (1st ed.). Routledge.
Lapping, C. (Ed.). (2020). *Freud, Lacan, Zizek and Education: Exploring Unconscious Investments in Policy and Practice*. Routledge.
Malabou, C. (2023). *Stop Thief! Anarchism and Philosophy*. Polity.
Meillasoux, Q. (2009). *After Finitude. An Essay on the Necessity of Contingency*. Bloomsbury.
Nobus, D. (2023). *Transformations of Lacan's Teaching and Institutional Transmissions from 1963 Till 1967*. Presented to *Lacan Salon*, 19 November. https://www.youtube.com/watch?v=L4a1gzDpz3g
Peim, N. (2001). The History of the Present: Towards a Contemporary Phenomenology of the School. *History of Education, 30*(2), 177–190. https://doi.org/10.1080/00467600010012454

Peim, N. (2012). The Big Other: An Offer You Can't Refuse—Or Accept, in Some Cases. Education as Onto-Theological Principle (Empire): An Anti-Manifesto. *Other Education, 1*(1), 226–238.

Peim, N. (2020). The Meaning of Life: The Ontological Question Concerning Education through the Lens of Catherine Malabou's Contribution to Thinking. *Educational Philosophy and Theory, 53*(10), 1011–1023.

Peim, N. (2022). *Rethinking the Politics of Education*. Routledge.

Peim, N., & Stock, N. (2022). Education after the End of the World. How Can Education Be Viewed as a Hyperobject? *Educational Philosophy and Theory, 54*(3), 251–262.

Roseboro, D. L. (2008). Jacques Lacan and Education. A Critical Introduction.

Srinivasan, A. (2021). *The Right to Sex*. Bloomsbury.

Stock, N. (2021). Darkness and Light: The Archetypal Metaphor for Education. *Educational Philosophy and Theory, 53*(2), 151–159.

Stock, N. (2023). My Teaching. Lacanian Reflections from the Classroom. *New Associations*, 40.

Stock, N. (2024). Classroom Architecture and the Gaze. Beyond the Panopticon. *Discourse: Studies in the Cultural Politics of Education, 45*(4), 521–535.

Taubman, P. (2012). *Disavowed Knowledge. Psychoanalysis, Education, and Teaching*. Routledge.

Webster, J. (2023). The Most Hysterical Psychoanalyst. *Journal of the American Psychoanalytic Association, 71*(5), 907–931.

Willis, P. (1977). *Learning to Labour: How Working Class Kids Get Working Class Jobs*. Columbia University Press.

Zupančič, A., & Terada, R. (2015). Sex, Ontology, Subjectivity: In Conversation with Alenka Zupančič. *Psychoanalysis, Culture and Society, 20*, 192–206.

CHAPTER 2

The Teacher

Abstract Developing the Real/Symbolic/Imaginary ontology of education outlined in chapter one, this chapter situates the figure of the teacher as a subject within that ontology. Initially, via the concept of *objet a*, the chapter explores Lacan's own allusions to teaching surrounding pedagogy, topics, and relationship with students. It discusses the formal aspects of Lacan's educational methods such as cartels and a new psychoanalytic school. The chapter then goes on to explain Lacan's figure of the split subject specifically as a teacher through the concept of the signifier. The teacher as a subject is further presented as the ego ideal/ideal ego figure found in Lacan's accounts of the Mirror Stage and the gaze, all of which contribute to constructing a particular form of subject found only in the space of the classroom.

Keywords Split subject • Signifier • objet a • Ego ideal • Ideal ego • Mirror stage • Gaze • Teacher • Student • Cartel • Classroom

I am going to try to speak to you…
—(Jacques Lacan, Seminar VII, p. 51)

© The Author(s), under exclusive license to Springer Nature Switzerland AG 2025

N. Stock, N. Peim, *The Lacanian Teacher*, The Palgrave Lacan Series, https://doi.org/10.1007/978-3-031-93018-8_2

Lacan as a Teacher

In rethinking educational ontology through the tripartite division of the Real, Symbolic and Imaginary, our particular focus is on the teacher-subject that resides in this space. To begin, we may consider their desires and fantasies. *What do you want?* (E, p. 690) is a fundamental question of the subject for Lacan. Putting this question to the teacher placed within the domain of the school, the space we take to be the paradigm institution of education, we may sketch out a basic Lacanian phenomenology of the teacher in relation to whatever we may find to be the 'object' that she operates in relation to.

For now, we might pause on Lacan as the very subject that we are interested in here, a teacher, in a teaching space, a 'school', with students. In the previous chapter we noted Lacan's numerous references to teaching (too numerous even to recount here in a book on education, though we quote many throughout). These pedagogical references refer to a range of qualities and aspects of teaching, but generally are laced with irony, and are 'inherently, interminably, self-critical' (Felman, 1982, p. 38), often mocking of the audience, and certainly challenge dominant assumptions about teaching and learning in everyday educational discourse. Many comments relate to the structure of Lacan's lessons. The seminars, for example, divided into different daily sessions, tend to be initiated with brief pedagogical reflections, usually through an effacement of the position of the teacher. In Seminar XXIII, a seminar given at the latter end of his career (1975–1976), Lacan begins one session by mocking his own teaching, claiming 'Things aren't going so well' (p. 62). This apparently throwaway line makes the important claim that teaching always falls short, that it can never go according to plan—something particularly subversive when we see this comment made as a reflection of his whole teaching career thus far, a retroactive move. Lacan simply and bluntly highlights a 'difficult thought for education to bear ... that thought and thinking are uncontrollable, radical and subversive' (Bibby, 2011, p. 114). Much earlier (1959–1960), in Seminar VII Lacan seems to be heading in this subversive direction, as he begins 'I am going to *try* to speak to you...' (p. 51, our emphasis)—another indication of the necessarily feeble venture of explaining something to the Other in the classroom. It seems as if this question of the 'you', a question for the teacher that is usually that of the student as the Other, the one who is taught, becomes more problematic for Lacan as his career goes on. 'I explain nothing' (XVI, p. 139), he says elsewhere. Indeed, in his move to university teaching later in life, he regularly problematises even the very possibility of a teachable Other—crystallised in his statement that he is 'talking to brick walls', 'speaking by [him]self' (BW, p. 80).

Similar statements are made much earlier, however. Many of Lacan's references to teaching are interwoven with notions of ignorance, both of the teacher and the student. Seminar II proposes that

> ...there is no true teaching other than the teaching which succeeds in provoking in those who listen an insistence-this desire to know which can only emerge when they themselves have taken the measure of ignorance as such-of ignorance inasmuch as it is, as such, fertile-in the one who teaches as well. (II, p. 271)

We will address the essential correspondence between knowledge and ignorance in Lacan's thought in the fourth chapter on pedagogy, but here we note the self-directed barbs at the ignorant educator. We see this early Lacanian teaching as a version of the provocateur without knowledge, a figure of knowing ignorance that reveals as much in his students, perhaps a repetition of the Socratic mode of teaching found in Plato's dialogues.

In other places, the barbs are directed towards the audience. 'I was hoping the room wasn't going to be so full' (XIII, p. 74) he says to a class full of attendees—a joke I'm sure many lecturers dream of being able to make these days. Similarly, in Seminar VIII, he says 'For many of you the enigma was so complete that people asked "What? What did he say? Do you know?"' (p. 135), highlighting both (mis)understanding and the Other's desire as aspects of his students' learning. Teaching is clearly replete with misunderstanding, but Lacan emphasises that this is fundamental to the space itself, not the journey towards understanding.

No more telling example of his musings on misunderstanding can be found than this, however, from Seminar XX: 'I dreamt last night that when I arrived, no one was here. That confirms the wishful character of the dream' (XX, p. 118). It appears that, whether ironically or not, the teacher's wish for Lacan is to not have to teach, or at least to not face anyone that demands to be taught. Contradictorily, he can only enjoy this joke by *having* students, as other, to make it to. Already we sense the Lacanian approach to teaching inflected with positional irony and beset with a desire to erase the wayward desire of the Other. We also must note that the dream as wish fulfilment—a typical Freudian trope—and the figure of the teacher are entangled. Teachers and dreamers are one and the same, suggesting the necessity of an engagement with fantasy when adumbrating the position of the teacher. Still, for Lacan this irony is coupled with the continued act of teaching new topics every year over three decades when he could of course have remained only a clinician. Something about teaching seduced Lacan, and even his expulsion from the International Psychoanalytic Institute could not curb his compulsion to continue.

Lacan's teaching quips are found elsewhere in his addresses to the immediate Other of the audience. Demands for questions and interruptions are regular: for example 'I would prefer it if someone asked a question. I said *a* question. I'm not asking for several' (XXIII, p. 110). Elsewhere, 'I would really like it if, from time to time, I had a response, even a protest' (XX, p. 83). Examples abound: it seems clear what Lacan wants from his audience is, partly, a protestation of his role as the master. This recurring gesture resonates with Lacan's observation of the 'passion for ignorance' he finds in clinical patients: a 'phrase to describe the way his patients seemed to do everything they could to avoid acknowledging the causes of their suffering, even though most—if not all—of them came to him claiming that they wanted to know what lay behind their pain' (Salecl, 2019, p. 44). What Lacan is touching on here is not simply a lack of knowledge, but a 'passion', an enjoyment found in the rejection of knowing. Clearly, this is what Lacan identifies in his students in many apparently throwaway jibes.

Seminar XX begins with Lacan addressing his audience explicitly in the role of teacher. Recognizing their presence in the space of a classroom in the guise of students, 'I am still (*'encore'*) here' (XX, p. 1) he declares with irony, musing perhaps on the remarkable number of years the seminars have been happening and on the continued interest from his audience. But this same interest is quickly satirised: 'What has worked in my favour for a while is that there is also on your part, in the great mass of you who are here, an "I don't want to know anything about it."' (p. 1). It is in this wanting not to know that they 'find themselves attached (*lies*) to me' (p. 1). These quips initiate many of the threads of the seminar: for example, the subject of knowledge and knowing and the concept of returns. However, what is most interesting, for us at least, is the relationship between teacher and student. Lacan proposes the reason they keep coming back year after year, validating his occupation of the space of the teacher, is not a lack of knowledge eagerly waiting to be supplemented. It is that they don't want to know. Their ignorance creates his relationship with them, a relationship that will also be troubled throughout our reading of Lacan's Seminar XX in Chap. 5 where we find echoes of an absence of a pedagogic relationship.

Later in the session, where Lacan claims that 'what constitutes the weight of my presence here—it's that you enjoy it' (p. 12), it would seem he falls into the same trap as any teacher, believing that enjoyment must be experienced by the student to allow the teacher to teach them. As Matthew Perry's Mr. Clark claims in the saccharine tv film *The Ron Clark Story* when his students destroy his classroom, 'I hoped we were really gonna have some fun this year'. Other teachers will often claim, 'If only they listened, they might enjoy themselves'. But Lacan offers a further, less subtle, subversion of his position: 'My sole presence is my stupidity' (p. 12). Lacan too participates in the stupidity of the learning relation—what else could it be? Only ever a series of half-saids and misunderstandings, the teaching relation demands that 'Stupidity nevertheless has to be nourished' (p. 14). Similar statements arise later in the seminar, especially in Lacan's discussion of learning development: 'Development is confused with the development of mastery' (p. 56). Mastery is a notoriously absurd aim for any Lacanian subject, something that will be obvious in our discussion of the subject in this chapter and in our description of knowledge in Chap. 4. Yet, mastery is prized and pursued in the path of education. The development of the student towards a mastery of their subject (and implicitly themselves as a subject) is a standard educational desideratum.

On a similarly troubling note for the conventional figure of the teacher, at the outset of Lacan's short lecture *The Place, Origin and End of My Teaching,* he initiates an attack on the dominant image of psychoanalysis in tandem with a meta-presentation of his perspective on teaching: 'I do not think I will give my teaching in the form of a pill; I think that would be difficult' (MT, p. 3). Lacan's view of his teaching, like his view of psychoanalysis, is that it is not easy to swallow like a pill. There is no condensed form that can be imbibed by his students, just as analysis cannot be a simple cure, if a cure at all (Reshe, 2023). If psychoanalysis resembles teaching, it is not like the staged, curricularised, target-driven, pill-like teaching we are so commonly invited to imagine, with its lesson plan, aims and staggered progression towards already determined learning outcomes. Lacan instead 'thought on stage, speaking extemporaneously often for an hour or more' (Webster, 2023, p. 908), resisting every instinct to plan and over-prepare. Rather, he read, he thought, and he free-associated on the stage of teaching, and spoke without a clear or intentional function (MT,

p. 5). Lacan takes the educational implications further, sarcastically claiming 'we are always a little cretinized because there is no escaping secondary school' (p. 74). School as cretinization, though not a phrase we would use, implies Lacan's distaste for the systems of institutionalised education, whether that be because of their pedagogical methods, curricula, or societal goals.

The function of the teacher is also faintly visible in Lacan's negative representation of 'the uncertainty that remains regarding the very end of analysis' (E, p. 191), something we might couple with the uncertainty of the end of education. Psychoanalysis is not a cure, in the medicalised sense of the eradication of symptoms and restoration to untroubled, smooth functioning. In *Negative Psychoanalysis for the Living Dead* (2023) Julie Reshe proposes a negative alternative to what she calls contemporary 'therapeutic culture' (p. 3). Seeing the positive as dishonest, suspicious of any idea that the ailing and the wounded are special cases, she asks: 'what if the whole world … is terminally sick with the same condition'? She identifies the 'omnipresent psychologization of society' as a misguided therapeutic turn seeking to invite preferably 'self-cure' while offering false remedial hope destined for disappointment (Reshe, 2023, pp. 3–5).[1] As we have stated in the first chapter, education follows signifying chains of cure, salvation, redemption. The ceaseless positivity, the upwards procession of education, a sort 'wishing people well' (MT, p. 10), a link between the '"good of all"' and 'the good of the individual' (p. 10) is a position Lacan consistently challenges. On one occasion, he goes so far as to identify a student as 'taking the piss' (p. 15) in calling him Jesus Christ, the primal figure of redemption. Messianism is precisely not the position Lacan believes his teaching (and thus analysis) might occupy.[2]

At stake in Lacanian questions of teaching, then, is not simply a question of ignorance and knowledge. There is something rather more fundamental to the experience. Teachers are regularly faced with the horror of

[1] Reshe, a self-professed Lacanian, sees the positive as dishonest. Suspicious of any idea that the ailing and the wounded are special cases, she identifies the 'omnipresent psychologization of society' as a therapeutic turn seeking to invite (preferably) 'self-cure' while offering false hope destined for disappointment (Reshe, 2023, p. 20).

[2] Though arguably the way Lacan has been positioned by many of his followers and readers is that of a Messianic figure. Even the most diligent reader, Derrida, can misread Lacan as a saviour figure who is therapeutically oriented. In Derrida's essay *For the Love of Lacan* (1998), still we find an adherence to the claim that Lacan demands 'apelike, orthodox' (p. 60) followers—a clear image of the writ of dogma.

the question of desire from their students. What do they want from me? This is felt most markedly on the first day of term standing in front of a new class as you babble about the syllabus, hoping this is what they want. Perhaps an icebreaker; they want to get to know each other? Or maybe just get straight into the curriculum? Cut the fluff: they don't really care about all that, do they? Maybe they don't care either way, and just want the bell to ring. This uncertainty can remain with some classes for whole terms, even a year, endlessly confronting the enigmatic desire of the Other.

The phenomenology of basic teaching relations is encapsulated in the singular question Lacan asks for in Seminar XXIII that we quoted earlier: 'I would prefer it if someone asked a question. I said *a* question' (XXIII, p. 110). This implies the need for the audience to formulate the question of their desire: what do they want from Lacan, the teacher? And is what they want what he wants? Though an unintended parallel made only from the translation, '*a* question' invokes the idea of the *objet a,* the object cause of desire. Objet a is, in Lacanian terms, a 'slippery' (VIII, p. 147) object, something that the subject encounters in the symbolic that charms them (p. 147). Anything we think we genuinely desire, be it a new fountain pen or a new way of life, is constituted in the realm of language while tethered to the Real desire of our unconscious. To offer an example, one might see an image of Edward Said, say, holding a Scheafer fountain pen. Via an Imaginary identification with the figure of the radical academic this object becomes desirable in the attempt to encapsulate this image. The pen becomes *objet a,* a fragment that one's desire can be invested in, but a desire that is really unknowable due to its unconscious corporeality. Certainly, there *is* a Real desire at play here, but that is not what the *objet a* is.

Lacan describes *objet a* via Plato's *Symposium* as the *agalma,* a small statue of a god—an object worthy of our desire, but the statue opens and contains within it jewels and metonymically signifies so much more that itself. Said's fountain pen has much the same effect, so that on obtaining it, we might find somewhere within our possession of it the jewels of being a radical academic. Lacan gives a similar example himself, where he recites a letter sent to him by some students. In the letter, they request Lacan send them some 'crafty tricks' for deploying his thought, along with one of his famous 'lovely bow ties' (XVI, p. 146). The ability to *be Lacan,* to occupy his position and do what he does, is imagined in donning the object that he is identified with. There is something ultimately uncanny (VIII, p. 147) about the *objet a* in this respect, as it occupies such a strong place of desire for us, and yet in obtaining it we brush up against its Real, usually finding it to be nothing more than trash. It is at once *so* vital to us and yet at the same time worthless. We see this in teaching all the time: where the teacher believes a new text, a new classroom gadget, a new syllabus, a new seating plan, a new head of department will complete their teaching and bring educational fulfilment. Once it becomes clear that these objects will not bring satisfaction, the teacher seeks a new desirable object once more.

Schools and Cartels

Though not our dominant concern, we might consider Lacan's engagement with the more formal aspects of education,[3] something that reveals other aspects of his view of the teacher. Despite being a vital figure in the teaching of analysts throughout the 1950s in the International Psychoanalytic Association (I.P.A.), he was 'excommunicated' (to use Lacan's own words in Seminar XI) from the I.P.A. after challenging some of their core dogmas. Lacan then formed new psychoanalytic schools to continue the radical reworking of Freud he had initiated in the 1950s. In 1964 (and again in 1980) Lacan founded a new school—a school in both senses of the word, a school of thought and an educational institution (albeit without a building) for the dissemination of knowledge. In this school, *L'Ecole Freudienne de Paris,* Lacan proposed structural formations with significant implications for the figure of the educator and the position they occupy. This transformation is particularly evident in his conception of 'the cartel', supposedly a structure that recentres desire and supplants the passion for ignorance found in most learning relationships. He described the cartel as follows:

> For the execution of the work, we shall adopt the principle of an elaboration supported in a small group. Each of these (we have a name to designate these groups) will be composed of three people at least, of five at most, four is the right measure. PLUS ONE charged with the selection, with the discussion and with the outcome to be reserved to the work of each.

[3] Those more familiar with Lacan's work might notice the omission of the four discourses found in Seminar XVII and its explicitly educational strand of 'university discourse'. Certainly some of the conclusions we have arrived at mirror Lacan's description of the university in this discursive formation, but we deliberately look elsewhere to the less commonly read aspects of Lacan regarding education. See Matthew Clarke's book *Lacan and Education Policy* (2019a) for an account of the four discourses in relation to contemporary education.

> After a certain period of functioning, the elements of a group will be invited to permute into another one. This office of directing will not constitute a fiefdom in which the service performed might be capitalised on to gain entry to a higher grade, and no one will have to regard himself as demoted by going back to the bottom rung of the work.
>
> For the reason that every personal enterprise will restore its author to the conditions of criticism and supervision to which any work to be undertaken will be submitted in the School. This in no way implies an inverted hierarchy, but a circular organisation whose functioning, easy to program, will be firmed up with experience. (FA, p. 1)

This is a radical reimagination of the structure of formal schooling so commonly found in the typical modern school, notably in its circular organisation with rotating group lead, its commitment to tasks selected by the group, its tight unit of the optimal four members. Though the figure of the plus one acts as the educator in the cartel as an overseer, there is the always possibility of their dethroning in a different cartel. As such, there is commonality certainly with Ivan Illich's deschooling model from 1970, in which networks of learners are set up with networks of experts, and one can move independently between the positions as one sees fit (Illich, 1970). But this horizontal form of education belies the function of the educator as Lacan clearly sees it. Though the school is reimagined, the educator is found more clearly in his position as the seminar instructor over his twenty-seven-year long delivery. As we have stated in Chap. 1, though we believe education to be an inherently irredeemable ontotheology,[4] there is still room for rethinking the figure of the teacher that exists within it—something we have shown Lacan does himself in his allusions to teaching. We have far from exhausted these educational traces in Lacan, but for now turn our attention more closely to the figure of the teacher as a subject under the Lacanian eye, and then consider the fantasies that substantiate such a figure.

[4] Ontotheology can be seen as '... our metaphysicians' ontological understandings of what entities are "as such" ground intelligibility from the inside out, while their theological understandings of the way in which the "totality" of beings exist simultaneously secure the intelligible order from the outside in' (Thomson, 2005).

The Teacher as a Subject and Their Signifiers

As we have raised in the previous chapter, the subject is central to Lacanian ontology—the being that is *in* the tripartite division of RSI. What is demotically referred to as an individual, a person, or a human being, Lacan refers to as the subject—the being created in and by language, 'the enunciating subject' (E, p. 800) who is both enunciated and who enunciates subjectivity. We are here interested in that subject who not only enunciates their subject-ness, but who is also enunciated by and through the signifier 'teacher'—an identification that once spoken becomes inhabited by and inhabits the subject, an identification that occurs by passing through a big language configuration, the big Other. As Lacan says, when I say who I am, 'I become incarnate, I crystalize' (VIII, p. 240). The speaking subject's enunciation of oneself as a subject, or indeed as 'a teacher', requires the use of a specific 'cluster' of already established and ordered signifiers from the big Other. Each subject is caught up in symbolic relations with this big Other, the very relations we explore in this book, particularly in our recount of the educational Symbolic order in the previous chapter.

These relations can be thought of in a simple way as 'one's relation to the Law, to the law laid down by one's parents' one's *teachers*, one's religion, one's country' (Fink, 1999, p. 33, our emphasis). The subject remains not so much directly controlled by these figures but entrammelled, caught up with them symbolically, no matter how "real" or not they might be. There is ambiguity in the subject's being subjected but it is also the first person 'I' that takes on the entrammelling subjectivation. No matter what they are, the subject defers to the big Other, and, as Fink makes clear in the previous quote, 'one's teachers', it is interesting that this big Other can be easily substituted for the signifier 'education'. Education is a 'big' subjectifier, as, at least since the mandatory education Forster Act of 1870 in the UK or other compulsory schooling policies elsewhere, we are all subjects of education required to give an account of ourselves as such. Though 'the educational Other' (Fink, 1999, p. 33) is not Real as such—it can't be—it remains a figure to which we who are embroiled in education defer and in turn act accordingly. It reverberates with the Real. These things that we do habitually in education are strongly tied to the logic and grammar of education that permeates every corner of it, whether this be in standard classroom pedagogy, educational research, governmental policy, media depiction, or even 'liberatory' methods. One cannot imagine a world where we do not educate, or prioritise education. In this disposition we defer to the big Other.

There is something about the teacher unlike other careers and professions that is particularly 'signifiery', closely attuned to the big Other. We might note how Lacan says 'There is no way of following me without passing through my signifiers, but to pass through signifiers involves the feeling of alienation that incites them to seek' (XI, p. 217). The student must pass through the teacher's signifiers (though of course said signifiers do not belong to the teacher; they derive from the big Other through the Symbolic of education). Assessment stands as an obvious example, where, whatever the subject, the student must conjure the correct formulation of signifiers to advance. Students must not only learn to repeat the signifiers of the teacher, mostly repetitions of the curriculum, but must also pass through the acceptance of the teacher: 'a good response!', 'wrong answer', 'could you expand on that for me?', 'tell your partner'. These pedagogic signifiers reaffirm the role of the teacher in the continuous assessment of the student, but they also alienate and split the student. This alienating or splitting is the process of having to 'be' someone only as a signifier, thus not quite what you think you are. Though student and teacher are adjured to believe this relation leads up the path to wholeness, it is rather the repetition of the splitting of the subject by the signifier. Most commonly, this happens through the 'binary signifier' (XI, p. 219), prevalent in the educational Symbolic order and indeed beyond it. Such binaries haunt the educational Symbolic: pass/fail, progress/regress, ignorant/enlightened, literate/illiterate, well-behaved/naughty; the list could go on. But the subject of education might see that 'beyond this signification, to what signifier—to what irreducible, traumatic, non-meaning—he is, as a subject, subjected' (p. 251). The teacher is subjected to these binaries, required to activate them in the language of the classroom.

Basil Bernstein's (1975) cogent sociology of education offers an interesting parallel here. The field of educational practices for Bernstein can be divided into 'classification' and 'framing' as axes of operation. The former refers to the systematized order of knowledge and the status positions that arise from it, a more or less stable ordering with determinate processes. The latter signifies the habitual practices, locations and identities at play in the delivery of the educational order. There is a dynamic relation between the two, but they both carry with them language uses that are specifically coded, and that make demands on the subjects of education to 'be' in a certain mode, as well as constantly making judgments about their position in the very hierarchical order of things. For Bernstein, code is critical in determining where you stand, in terms of 'orientation to meaning': and this applies to the occupant of the most elevated academic position as well as to the most abject educational reject. In addition, Bernstein indicates how social identity gets differentially recoded through education to reproduce social inequalities that arise from the social 'division of labour of educational knowledge' (1975, p. 88).

The Lacanian perspective clearly chimes with Bernstein and a number of powerful sociological and theoretical strands. In the school's (education's) obsession with ranking and ordering, the teacher and the pupil are locked into an interplay of the subject's sense of self that activates the production of signifiers of difference. The logic of assessment positions all in a relation organized by what Heidegger has referred to as 'technological enframing' (1977), the imposition of a process of ranking and ordering designed to render beings knowable and useful, inscribed into judgments of relative value. These involve Imaginary identifications for Lacan, systems of *méconnaissance* that generate the feeling of relationality in the classroom through signifiers of ranking. Lacan gives the example of a child attempting to find some sense of identification of themselves whilst playing a game of odds and evens. In 'an internal imitation of his opponent's attitudes' (E, p. 43), believing they have understood the rules of the game, they think they find an other that gives them identity as a winner (or indeed as a loser). Lacan also discusses Freud's myth of the primal horde found in *Totem and Taboo* (SE XIII) in a similar way, where 'rivalry among the brothers, is the basis for identification' (p. 95). In both examples, we believe we identify with another if we are ranked above or below them, after all, but even more so if we are the one who is able to do the ranking.

In the contemporary context, this process of ranking and ordering, managed formally by institutions of inspection, differentially defines the performative value of teachers and schools. Universities, in turn, are not immune to this process most often experienced by teachers and students as the essence of the educational experience, despite lingering fantasies of a pure education devoid of, or somehow outside of, assessment. The reform-hungry teacher, strongly activated by an ethic of social justice, may enter the educational scene with intentions of rising above the 'anti-educational' practices of assessment, but, by force of the Symbolic order, is obliged to become its agent, constantly making judgments and subjecting pupils to the assessment order. Although this dimension of education has long been articulated, and has never been circumvented, the discourse of equality prevails in educational institutions, often among educational professionals who must either subscribe to a misplaced faith in meritocracy or who must constantly long for the day when the demons of assessment are exorcised from the educational scene (Allen, 2011, 2014). What education would look like, were this to happen, and how it would be motivated, remains to be seen (or not). Questions concerning assessment and its role in social injustice mostly, rooted in social class biases, cannot be addressed by those destined to enact its procedures. Despite decisive—and largely uncontested—demonstrations of education's vital role in reproducing social class inequalities, these perspectives must be foreclosed (Reay, 2017).

As we will discuss in the final chapter, this relationship between the signifier and the subject in the classroom will have bearings on modes of enjoyment, especially if we seek new ones. But it does other things too: the alignment between teaching and passing through the signifier is how education reaps its subjects, cuts them in half with the signifying chains that make education what it is. The cut 'carves up (divides) the body image and thus drives the subject to seek its being beyond that which its image presents to it; it causes the subject always to find in its image something lacking' (Britzman, 2015, pp. 50–51). This cut that drives the subject to see itself as inherently lacking is mostly disavowed, especially by teachers lured by an ideal of wholeness by the Symbolic order of education. Becoming a teacher is a signifier of having become educated to the point of being able to educate others, a process magnified in academia by the granting of honorifics for the 'most' educated subjects. But as the subject strives, consciously or unconsciously, to prevent itself from confronting its inherent lack, it must avoid the sense of not being whole and of not being master in one's own house. To reiterate, it is in the pursuit of education that avowal of the subject's lack is elided.

Students are presumed by teachers to be (albeit differentially) on the path to wholeness, completion, in becoming educated whether formally through the signifiers of grades, or more abstractly through the master signifier of education 'itself'. The model student in turn believes that they can obtain completion as a subject by achieving education. The discipline of philosophy of education that we think would offer alternatives has almost universally disavowed this essential relation of lack that is so central to the Lacanian project. Thus a retreading of the philosophy of education, through the Lacanian mode of thinking, is so important in this book.

Subjects and Subjects

A curious resonance exists in the English language between the centrality of the subject in Lacanian thought and 'subjects' as fundamental to teaching. There is a powerful, and largely unexplored correspondence, between these registers. Subjects in schools allow for the 'division of the school day, the movement of students', they designate 'the labour of teachers' and classify 'forms of knowledge' (Britzman, 1991, p. 35)—all critical parts of the disciplinary apparatus of schooling discussed in the first chapter. But more interesting in the Lacanian vision is the way subjects in schools are not only knowledge subjects, but also subjects as in people who identify with their subjects.

To restate what we said at the start of this section, the subject is incapable of enunciating themself without the invocation of signifiers from a pool of already-existing language, a pool that is the (essentially substanceless) form of the big Other. The Lacanian psychoanalyst Stijn Vanheule neatly summarises this process of subjectivation, noting that all of us are unconsciously responding to a set of existential questions and conflicts that must be articulated in the confrontation with life's daily encounter with the existential challenge. As such, we must speak: 'Answers must be formulated' (Vanhelue, 2023, p. 77), to fabricate a sense of meaning and purpose. Such answers must use signifiers; but these signifiers will always be insufficient to the task. We might bear witness to this process in the Symbolic division between being a student and teacher, or through being in school and the 'real world'. To proclaim oneself as 'a teacher' is to invoke a—heavily loaded—signifier from the realm of language so to substantiate oneself as subject. The specific teacher is not the signifier, of course; they have a dimension of the Real that is not just language. They remain curiously alienated from it, divided from themselves, but governed by the signifier's movement as part of the Symbolic order they have drawn it from. It is what allows the subject to participate and make sense of what engulfs them. Vanheule uses another example about teaching to substantiate this claim: 'Thanks to the signifier "lecturing", I can situate myself as a "speaker" and the others as "audience", which organizes my mental representations' (p. 79). What is particularly interesting about teaching in this instance is that, in line with Vanheule's conceptualization of the subject as determined by a demand to use signifiers to respond to existential questions of the unconscious, teachers often act as the treasure trove (and guardians) of signifiers for the student: another agalma to be desired. Any student that finds themself in the questioning of their being must seek answers, and so often the teacher must pose as holding the answer to the questions through ingratiating a new realm of signifiers with which to respond. And of course, 'no signifier can answer exclusively' (p. 77) these questions.

The use of subjects in schools function in a similar way: if you ask group of students (or indeed teachers) what 'the subject' is, they of course respond with English, Maths, Sociology, Law, etc. and in the strange (classification obsessed) environment of the school, students often identify themselves through their subjects—'I am an English student', 'Well, I am a Biology student.' This is even more pronounced among teachers who regularly must identify themselves through the question 'what do you teach?' or cite their subject when telling people outside of teaching what they do. Yet what these subjects confront with each other is only their subjects. As Lacan famously says, the signifier is 'that which represents a subject for another signifier' (XI, p. 207). When we encounter another, we are both entrammelled in the signifying chain that speaks us. We cannot appear in the guise of 'authentic' selves, but as two signifiers representing one another to one another. The signifier does designate a subjective Real that pre-exists its formulation in language, giving rise to a splitting of the subject. In this way Lacan again aligns himself with Bernstein (1975) for whom identity is always caught up in specific modes of speech that are coded according to (for example) social class differences that determine a specific orientation to meaning. Lacan is going beyond class, however, to the ontological level of our subjectivity.

Much like Heidegger's signifier of ~~Being~~ under erasure ['sous rature']—a self-effacing signifier as Derrida (1976) notes, Lacan continues this ontologically unstable being by presenting the subject through the symbol of a barred S ($). This bar is important, for it signifies the divided nature of the subject who speaks itself as a subject. Essential elements of Freudian psychoanalysis give weight to this Lacanian division, including the divide between conscious and unconscious, id/ego and super-ego, thus defining the subject from the get-go as unable to know dimensions of themself with any stable, rational confidence. Even in Freudian parlance, the teacher is never going to be that figure of mastery demanded in the Symbolic of education. Freud also speaks of the early severing between the baby and the mother's breast, a primal trauma intensified by Kristeva (1984) in her assertion of the abjection of the subject through the very necessitated act of being birthed thus (r)ejected by the mother.

Though these divisions are important and remind us of the fundamentally wounded or severed nature of the subject, Lacan's key insight is that the subject is 'barred', cut or divided by the signifier we spoke of previously. To speak is to efface oneself. Enlightenment philosophy and its pervasive influence on commonsense belief see the human as at least potentially full, able to be complete. We can become finished individuals, acting in control of ourselves, whether selfish or altruistic. But for Freud in his discoveries of the unknowability of the unconscious and the implacability of the drive, this image of 'man' is unsettled and disturbed. Teachers, like any other subject, are divided and incomplete, always already lacking, constantly seeking to plug the gap and always failing, and yet always talking more and more, further cutting.

What's more, the division of the subject also occurs because each subject must say what she wants. Desire, here different from demand (E, p. 689), like the need to be heard and understood by the students, is found through signifiers (p. 689). We should recall that signifiers are drawn from the big Other, here perhaps the educational big Other. Thus, if you ask teachers what they want, in the peculiar world of the school they often draw on signifiers like 'helping students get good grades', 'getting them into university', 'helping them develop a love learning', and so on. Though many of these answers are often easily explained by the so-called neoliberal agenda that haunts contemporary education, the Lacanian dimension allows us to explore the structure of education beyond the alleged neoliberal enclosure (Clarke, 2021). While the drive to achieve good grades and university admissions may indicate a relatively recent instrumentalization of education (at least according to some), many teachers invoke a multifaceted ethical dimension to their work, making claims to educate the student in some more far-reaching, perhaps even redemptive sense. Many communicate a positive sense of the governmental force of schooling as essential to good social order in the widest sense, indicating their attachment to a social educational ethic. Undoubtedly, this ethical dimension (whereby the self is attached to a positive collective project) is where the enjoyment for many teachers lies and is perhaps automatically caught up in the discourses of teaching. Believing themselves agents of positive change for their charges, and for the world in turn, of course presupposes an alignment with the desires of the Other. Just as in the prior description of the barred subject, such teacher enjoyment is in tune with the logic of lack that can't be closed so that enjoyment accrues from the inevitably failing attempt, from the suspension of the desired final outcome.

The Gaze and the Mirror

A key part of the process of subjectivation is the gaze, another central concept in both Lacan and certain analyses of education. Often, the gaze is conflated with Foucauldian panoptic surveillance (Copjec, 2015; Stock, 2024). The image of the panopticon that Michel Foucault presents has dominated certain critical educational discourses. From this perspective, the classroom is imagined as a functional site of surveillance where bodies are managed for modes of governance and self-governance, ideally resulting in the production of the self-managing individual (Foucault, 1991). The gaze at play is both invisible and omnipresent—internalised by the student and inherent in the structuration of the classroom. But the Lacanian gaze is akin to the gaze we find in mirrors and screens—the gaze that looks back at us. The concept of the gaze gets developed throughout Lacan's career and is modified at times, but its origins are in the famous Mirror Stage. The mirror stage is a developmental event of the ego, both metaphorical and literal, that a child goes through when they see themselves in a mirror as an autonomous being. I lift my arm, and the being in the mirror lifts its arm. I frown, and the being in the mirror frowns. Cause and effect and control of the body induce a moment of subjectification for the child who perceives a fully formed self. This engagement with their 'specular image' is a 'jubilatory' moment (X, p. 32). The child apprehends their ego, or *Ich* in the original German, in the mirror, in what is really the ego-ideal, a version of themselves from the perspective of a total view where the 'fragmented body' (E, p. 97) appears as a completed entity. For Lacan, what this stage presents is a myth of integrated wholeness. What is missing from the image seen in the mirror is the Other that put them there and on which they depend, such as a parent (X, p. 32). But equally it occludes the unconscious dimensions of their subjectivity. They imagine themselves to be whole when they engage with this mirror image, a promise of a future of perfection and control over themselves (Herbert, 2012, p. 23) but really they are lacking. There is a gap between the image that the subject has of themselves and the subject. The mediated image framed by the screen-like surface of the mirror confirms that our sense of completion is only to be achieved virtually: 'caught in the butterfly net of culture' as Catherine Belsey has it (2004, p. 101).

The mirror is not just a simple reflection, just as a picture is not simply a picture of something outside of and different from oneself. The image seen in the mirror is that of oneself as a character or figure, an individual that one believes an Other may see. The 'mirror is conceived of as a screen' (Copjec, 2015, p. 16) and the subject sees themselves being seen. The implication is that the image of the self that looks back at the subject, the thing that sees me, the gaze, creates a fantasy akin to that of a film, of a complete subject embedded in a more or less coherent narrative. The Imaginary wholeness granted to the subject by the gaze by looking in the mirror echoes the end point of the most prevalent discourses around teaching, particularly in relation to claims of developmental logic of children through their education. This logic is inherently psychologistic, inflected with the 'overwhelming influence of Jean Piaget' (Johnson, 2014, p. 2) and his theory of cognitive development, even if there are some other interlocutors being installed in English education such as Baddeley (1992) and his storage memory model alongside a reduced interpretation of Vygotsky's 'Zone of Proximal Development' (1978) (all discussed further in Chap. 4).

Relations between teachers and learners cannot be reduced to a merely functional positioning. For one thing, the teacher demands the gaze of the student to subjectivate them as a teacher. If the student is not looking, they are not in the picture: that is, teaching and learning cannot take place. Solzhenitsyn (1999) refers to this visual excitement of the classroom for the teacher, demanding attention, demanding some obeisance to the order of knowledge the teacher's ego (ideal) wants to sustain. As Bibby notes, 'gazing out of a window can be highly productive … a threat to the teacher's authority' (2011, p. 114). All such gestures towards deconstruction of the authority structure of the classroom, however, must temporarily, at least, forget the intensely loaded Symbolic and Imaginary framing of educational spaces. Lacan says, 'The gaze I encounter … is not a seen gaze, but the imagined by me in the field of the Other' (XI p. 84); and differently, as Anna Herbert notes, 'I see you seeing me, I interpret your desire yet all this happens unconsciously' (2012, p. 22). Both the development of the child and the position of the teacher are complicated by the Lacanian perspective on the psycho-social architecture of the classroom. The gaze the student experiences (of the teacher) carries a disciplinary component, echoing the fantasy of what the Other believes is desired to be seen. But this gaze is not simply disciplinarian; it may activate love, hate, fear, whatever fantasy may have been unconsciously constructed that the teacher expresses and that the teacher in turn constructs for themselves in the light of the gaze they feel.

This of course works in reverse too, as the gaze sustains the internalised punishment, or masochism, of the teacher. As Lacan says, the 'ascetic who flagellates himself does it for a third party' (XI, p. 183), that is, the gaze of the Other present in the space and 'Things' (p. 109) of the classroom. Such an irony that the students believe it is the teacher who is the holder of this gaze and, some, studiously flagellate themselves for better grades (or not) or approval, whilst really it is the teacher who is the one tortured by the gaze. The gaze always asks "what do you want" of the subject—we are made by what we think the Other wants, though of course this is something we cannot know.

We might find examples of the gaze in the actions of a teacher who deems the action they performed as contrary to their own image of their self. Many teachers, ourselves included, do not care about lateness. What does it matter if the student misses part of the lesson when you have let go of the fantasy that you (or the lesson) make such a difference? And yet, still you find yourself put out by their tardiness, ready to challenge them with another sarcastic comment when they eventually saunter into the classroom. This process indicates the subjectivating nature of the gaze, where we see ourselves in the picture that we thought we had transgressed. Britzman gives us another similar example in her study of student teachers undergoing the process of learning to teach. One trainee, who opposes discipline and even lacks faith in the school system, finds herself saying '"Matt, come back here"' (1991, p. 86) as one student walks away from her mid-dialogue. Tellingly, she says '"I don't know where it came from"' (p. 86). Such is the nature of the image we hold of ourselves in the mirror. This teacher, just like the authors of the book, saw themselves as anti-authoritarian. And yet, in that classroom space, one does what a teacher does … and often with some enjoyment.

The Teacher's Ego

The Mirror Stage and the gaze are tied to the process of ego formation, or as would be more precise in Lacanian theory, ego destitution. Immediately this is radical for thinking through education, posing the question that does the identification that happens in the classroom above "make" subjects or does it destitute them? The subject is caught up between the two. We might look at how in early stages of Lacanian theory, the ego itself is the product of a form of misrecognition, *méconnaissance* (I, p. 167). It is the specular image of the self that furnishes the ego with the illusion of unity. This specular image, however, lies outside of the self, and remains always ideal. The ideal of unity is the necessary condition of perception even while it constantly eludes us. Its absence engenders anxiety: the anxiety of dissolution. Hence it cannot be internalized and adopted as a consistent unifying principle of integrity. In later work (E, p. 95), Lacan expands this idea of the ideal ego in relation to the Freudian analysis of the narcissistic, self-aggrandizing ego. The synthesis arrived at represents the ego as having its basis in both the narcissistic idealization and the specular image of unity. As Žižek says, 'imaginary identification is identification with the image in which we appear likeable to ourselves, with the image representing "what we would like to be"' (1989, p. 174).

The specular image thus represents the self but also the self in the *position* of the other who gazes at the self that we might find some identification with. Again, the teacher who finds themselves shouting about lateness or anxious about inspection, even if they have consciously rejected these minor laws of teaching, still identifies with the onlooker, be it the inspector, the student, or the big Other of education itself. The imaginary identification of the self with the ideal self is always already structured by a splitting—the teacher I want to be and the teachers I identify with in my act of teaching (a range of which will be explored in the next chapter on fantasy). This externalized, imaginary self is for the self an object of desire, the object the subject wants to be: the unitary, complete integrated self. If the teacher *finds* themselves being a certain way, then on some level this a self they desire. At the same time, this effect of projection makes a demand upon the self. In so far as the image represents the ideal self, it inhabits the self as an ideal in a narcissistic love relation. This ideal ego becomes in effect an imaginary other facing us as our 'proper' selves (Žižek, 1989, pp. 105–114).

Imaginary identification is not simply the desire to resemble or to occupy the place of a desired object: it is to fulfil an ideal on behalf of a perception of the gaze or desire of the other. Every attempt to realign the self or the ego to a Symbolic ideal is structured by a sense of enacting that ideal role or mode of being on behalf of another. This image of the gaze of the other is pivotal for the identification of the teacher with the signifier teacher. The subject as depicted in the mirror stage sees himself through the ego ideal: 'It is in the field of the Other … a major stage of identification is established … idealization, ego ideal' (XI, p. 256). The fully formed individual, one who knows, one who is complete and thus not lacking, is implicated in the gaze of the Other that is present in the image. Take for example this passage from Karl Ove Knausgaard's epic of autofiction *My Struggle*:

> I was after enrichment. And what enriched me while reading Adorno, for example, lay not in what I read but the perception of myself while I was reading. I was someone who read Adorno! And in this heavy, intricate, detailed, precise language whose aim was to elevate thought ever higher, and where every full stop was set like a mountaineer's cleat, there was something else, this particular approach to the mood of reality, the shadow of these sentences, which could evoke in me a vague desire to use the language with this particular mood on something real, on something living. (Knausgaard, 2013, p. 295)

The subject reading Adorno (or maybe even Lacan…) does so not (only) for the enrichment of the language available in the text, but rather for the being-a-reader-of-Adorno—the perception of oneself that must be the sort of the person who is Adornian, who has Adornian critiques. Much like the teacher described previously, the subject of the teacher is drawn, initially, from a faith in identification with the signifier "teacher" drawn from the big Other, existing in the symbolic. But by 'clinging to the reference-point of him who looks at him in the mirror, the subject sees appearing, not his ego ideal, but ideal ego, that point at which he desires to gratify himself in himself' (XI, p. 257). The ideal ego is ideal 'in the sense in which one says that a car is an ideal car. It is not a car's ideal, nor is it the dream of a car when it is all by itself in the garage—it is a truly good and solid car' (VIII, p. 333) The teacher might position themselves this way, as the ideal ego for a student to obtain, an ego worthy of an ideal.

Just to complicate things further, the ideal ego is distinguished from the ego-ideal (E, p. 562). Where the ideal ego has as its reference point in the other (self as other) who we wish to identify with, the ego-ideal is based on the idealized image of unity, but not so much in the Imaginary register as in relation to the Symbolic register. It is 'symbolic identification, identification with the very place *from where* we are being observed, *from where* we look at ourselves so that we appear to ourselves likeable, worthy of love' (Žižek, 1989, p. 174). For Lacan, the ego-ideal occurs in the reign of the signifier: it occurs where there is identification with the other as other in idealized form—with parents, their substitutes or with collective ideals or ideal forms in the domain of the Symbolic (Althusser, 1971; Butler, 1997, pp. 25–38, E, pp. 562–565). In education, this is a standing in relation to its ideal form, to its standards of perfection and completeness. We can easily recall the disgraced Mr. Keating at the close of *Dead Poets Society*. Despite his shame, 'the boys stand on their desks to salute Keating and the vision of education he has presented' (Clarke, 2019b, p. 190). Symbolically, Keating represents the ultimate agent of change, the 'spiritual leader' (p. 190), the all-loving father, that the teacher is demanded to identify with.

Being beyond the self and representing the image of completeness or perfection the ego-ideal is insatiably demanding, omnipotent. In Lacan's rewriting of Freud, the ego-ideal becomes the essential principle of social identity. In the context of the school, the teacher is subjected to the demand of the ego-ideal in a range of ways, through an array of practices formal and informal. Initially, there is the intricately specified order of competences the student teacher must answer to. Beyond that there is the constant reiteration of what it means to conduct oneself in a 'professional' manner, to be a teacher in accordance with a proper order of being: say, returning one's register on time, reading the daily bulletin to tutees, ensuring that school uniform requirements are being adhered to, finishing one's reports on time and appropriately, delivering the curriculum with verve and according to the letter of the syllabus, supporting one's colleagues and so on. In the case of the ego-ideal, there is little need for the explicit reiteration of these demands: they are to be experienced as written into the order of things, the symbolic order of the school regime. And, of course, this regulatory function of the ego-ideal is by no means restricted to the school. The educator is haunted by this figure of its own projection in whatever context.

We might finish by briefly mentioning a figure that Lacan describes to encapsulate the idealised teacher, what he calls the *sujet supposé savoir* (S.s.S.), the 'subject supposed to know' (XI, p. 232). It is fairly well trodden in educational theory that makes use of Lacan (Felman, 1982; Jay, 1987; Britzman, 2015), thus we will not spend long on it. Still, it is a figure who encapsulates the question: What happens when we think we have all the signifiers? The S.s.S. is easy to see in the clinical encounter, where a person suffering with some neurotic episode, say, seeks therapy so that a professional can tell them what is wrong with them. What happens in the psychoanalytic encounter is of course not therapeutic, as the analyst actually knows nothing of the analysand on their couch. It is only the analysand who knows, but at the same time they do not know due to the unconscious nature of their neurosis.

Such a figure is easily transposed into the classroom: students enter expecting to learn the answers from the teacher. No teacher, nor as Lacan says, the 'psychoanalyst, can claim to represent … a corpus of absolute knowledge' (XI, p. 232). But for both teaching and psychoanalysis to function, the student must believe that there is just such a subject who is supposed to know. They must know what is needed to pass the exam, to hit high grades, to improve the work, to be educated. They must know the correct interpretation of *Macbeth,* or the solution to an algebraic equation. Usually, S.s.S. is invoked in educational circles to challenge 'spoon-feeding', giving students the answer to exams in easily consumable portions or 'pill[s]' (MT, p. 3), but there is something more far-reaching about S.s.S. that challenges the position of an educator at all, in a far-reaching way, not just in terms of producing answers to exam questions.

It is common parlance in teaching these days to claim that one does not have to occupy such a position. Indeed, the enlightened modern educator will claim it doesn't matter if you don't know the answer to a student's question. You just need to be able to guide students towards it, suggest approaches, perhaps, or provide materials for independent learning. This pedagogical assumption is patently disavowed when a student asks a question the teacher does not know the answer to. Particularly in lesson observations, teachers are visibly shaken, students visibly unimpressed—an anxiety haunts the scene of any encounter with the fragility of the ego. The Symbolic structure of the space demands that there is someone who knows in the classroom, in the lecture theatre, and it shouldn't be the student or the search engine. It is as though the enlightened teacher must pose as the one who suspends occupying the role of S.s.S. in order to maintain the fiction that the student might also come to occupy that very position should they persist with their self-driven pursuit, even while the teacher assumes the pose of the one who does occupy the role of S.s.S., albeit implicitly.

What's more, students will often, by force of Symbolic habit as it were, credit the teacher as being the bearer of knowledge. At times, this attribution can spill outside of the subject of the subject and into questions about life in general: 'This isn't a question about the test, but I was wondering if you could tell me what I should do about my brother?' For the teacher it is often especially enjoyable when students begin asking how they should live their lives enabling the teacher to dispense pearls of wisdom beyond the confines of the curriculum. But what must be made clear is that 'As soon as the subject who is supposed to know [*S.s.S*] exists ... there is transference' (XI, p. 232). What this means is, as soon as such a pedagogic relationship exists, the disorderliness of the unconscious of both teacher and student starts to fire around the classroom. It is in this disorder that we find the Real of pedagogy, something we will examine in Chap. 4.

In the clinical encounter, Lacan notes that the patient seeks the S.s.S. but also hold onto its inverse, the passion for ignorance. Despite seeking therapy, when confronted with their unconscious desires and traumatic histories, they have a 'desire to ignore' (Felman, 1982, p. 40). It is too painful, after all, to encounter who we are beyond the ideal image in the mirror. This passion for ignorance may be transposable to the kind of classroom encounter where students are regularly maligned for not wanting to learn. This seems low hanging fruit, a cliché of teacher discourse, projecting an image of the 'learner' (child, pupil, student) that is constructed in relation to the ideal ego of the teacher. Surely, such passion for ignorance only holds true if we believe that education is Real in its pursuit of knowledge, that the teacher stands securely in the position of S.s.S. and that the curriculum is exactly as it ought to be? But Felman (1982) and Britzman (2015) both indicate and illustrate that the teacher is equally prone to a resistance to pedagogy that can take a maddening dynamic like that of the students' resistances to learning. Teachers may well get set in their ways and refuse to learn 'new' pedagogies as ways of engaging with their classes. This is certainly true in an Imaginary sense, but we are more interested here in the fantasy image of the teacher and the mythical pedagogical relation demanded by the passion for ignorance. Over the next three chapters, we will examine these more closely.

References

Others

Allen, A. (2011). Michael Young's the Rise of the Meritocracy: A Philosophical Critique. *British Journal of Educational Studies, 59*(4), 367–382.

Allen, A. (2014). *Benign Violence: Education in and Beyond the Age of Reason.* Palgrave Macmillan.

Althusser, L. (1971). Ideology and Ideological State Apparatuses. In L. Althusser (Ed.), *Lenin and Philosophy and Other Essays.* Monthly Review Press.

Baddeley, A. (1992). Working Memory. *Science, 255*(5044), 556–559.
Belsey, C. (2004). *Culture and the Real: Theorizing Cultural Criticism* (1st ed.). Routledge.
Bernstein, B. (1975). *Class, Codes and Control: Towards a Theory of Educational Transmission, Volume 3.* Routledge.
Bibby, T. (2011). *Education—An 'Impossible Profession'? Psychoanalytic Explorations of Learning and Classrooms.* Routledge.
Britzman, D. (1991). *Practice Makes Practice: A Critical Study of Learning to Teach.* SUNY Press.
Britzman, D. (2015). *A Psychoanalyst in the Classroom.* SUNY Press.
Butler, J. (1997). *Excitable Speech: A Politics of the Performative.* Routledge.
Clarke, M. (2019a). *Lacan and Education Policy. The Other Side of Education.* Bloomsbury.
Clarke, M. (2019b). Education beyond Reason and Redemption: A Detour Through the Death Drive. *Pedagogy, Culture & Society, 27*(2), 183–197.
Clarke, M. (2021). *Education and the Fantasies of Neoliberalism: Policy, Politics and Psychoanalysis* (1st ed.). Routledge.
Copjec, J. (2015). *Read My Desire. Lacan Against the Historicists.* Verso.
Derrida, J. (1976). *Of Grammatology* (G. C. Spivak, Trans.). Johns Hopkins University Press.
Derrida, J. (1998). *Resistances of Psychoanalysis.* Stanford University Press.
Felman, S. (1982). Psychoanalysis and Education: Teaching Terminable and Interminable. *Yale French Studies, 63*, 21–44.
Fink, B. (1999). *A Clinical Introduction to Lacanian Psychoanalysis: Theory and Technique.* Harvard University Press.
Foucault, M. (1991). *Discipline and Punish. The Birth of the Prison.* Penguin.
Heidegger, M. (1977). *The Question Concerning Technology, and Other Essays.* Harper & Row.
Herbert, A. (2012). Pedagogy and the Gaze. In B. Bergstedt, A. Herbert, & A. Kraus (Eds.), *Initiating Learning* (pp. 19–34). Waxmann Verlag.
Illich, I. (1970). *Deschooling Society.* Marion Boyars Publishers Ltd.
Jay, G. S. (1987). The Subject of Pedagogy: Lessons in Psychoanalysis and Politics. *College English, 49*(7), 785–800.
Johnson, T. R. (2014). *The Other Side of Pedagogy: Lacan's Four Discourses and the Development of the Student Writer.* SUNY Press.
Knausgaard, K. O. (2013). *A Death in the Family: Book 1—My Struggle.* Vintage Publishing.
Kristeva, J. (1984). *Revolution in Poetic Language.* Columbia University Press.
Reay, D. (2017). *Miseducation: Inequality, Education and the Working Classes* (1st ed.). Bristol University Press.
Reshe, J. (2023). *Negative Psychoanalysis for the Living Dead. Philosophical Pessimism and the Death Drive.* Palgrave Macmillan.

Salecl, R. (2019). Coul Ignorance be Bliss? *RSA Journal, 165*(4), 42–44.
Solzhenitsyn, A. (1999). *The Gulag Archipelago, 1918–1956*. Harvill.
Stock, N. (2024). Classroom Architecture and the Gaze. Beyond the Panopticon. *Discourse: Studies in the Cultural Politics of Education, 45*(4), 521–535.
Thomson, I. (2005). *Heidegger on Ontotheology* (1st ed.). Cambridge University.
Vanhelue, S. (2023). Conceptualizing and Treating (Manic-Depressive) Psychosis. In D. Hook & S. Vanheule (Eds.), *Lacan on Depression and Melancholia* (pp. 76–86). Routledge.
Vygotsky, L. S. (1978). *Mind in Society: The Development of Higher Psychological Processes*. Harvard University Press.
Webster, J. (2023). The Most Hysterical Psychoanalyst. *Journal of the American Psychoanalytic Association, 71*(5), 907–931.
Žižek, S. (1989). *The Sublime Object of Ideology*. Verso.

CHAPTER 3

Fantasies of Teaching

Abstract The world of the teacher as a subject is substantiated by examining a range of fantasies that hover in the educational imaginary. Drawing on film, policy, and anecdotes, the authors explore the fantasies of being 'born to teach', 'making a difference', being 'subject specialists' or intellectuals, and educating in a sadistic mode 'by any means necessary'. The fantasies are then depicted as an enactment in the classroom through a phenomenology of the mundane teacher. Recognising their own fantasies, the authors recount personal histories of their paths into teaching and beyond, with a concluding section that analyses the sort of subjects they imagined themselves to be as teachers.

Keywords Fantasy • Education policy • Film • Sadism • Phenomenology • Teacher • Anxiety • Wholeness • Student • English teacher

...he snips into teachings, he does something analogous to collage.
—(Jacques Lacan, Seminar X, p. 172)

© The Author(s), under exclusive license to Springer Nature Switzerland AG 2025

N. Stock, N. Peim, *The Lacanian Teacher*, The Palgrave Lacan Series, https://doi.org/10.1007/978-3-031-93018-8_3

Fantasy

What do you think of when you think of a teacher? Perhaps, you find in the realm of your Imaginary, a cocktail, 'collage' (X, p. 172) or 'bric-a-brac' (III, p. 155) of assorted images, ideas and outlines. Likely, at the forefront, if you are a teacher, is the image of yourself in the classroom (or at least the teacher in the classroom you hope people see). But even if you are a teacher, this might only be a minor aspect of the image. There will be traces of what you have been told a teacher is, a telling that comes from the bombardment of media texts and images, the formation of teacher aims and standards in educational policy, the misshapen memories we have of school. Some are openly fictionalised narratives that include teachers as both major and minor characters, whilst others are more documentarian representations that aspire to capture the 'reality' of the teacher.

There are of course a range of stipulations, signifiers of competence and proficiency, that surround the image of a teacher. In our UK context alone, there are numerous official frameworks defining the qualities and competences that project the image of the credentialed teacher.[1] Official projections may be supplemented by invocations of family members who are teachers or who, like that wise grandparent epitomize the teacher. Everyone, of course, has *that* teacher, the one who inspired them, who gave them a passion for their subject, who was amazing to be taught by, who controlled the class like the conductor of an orchestra, made effortless puns and gags. This fantastic teacher may not, in any real sense, have existed, but in the powerful narrativizing force of memory, that teacher may become a dominant image attached to the signifier of teacher. Lacan makes clear that the teacher does exactly this in their desire to teach (X, p. 172), and of course fantasy is vital for any subject. Only, Lacan notes that teachers are too concerned with the 'join' (p. 172) of these different shreds—too determined to make it a complete ego ideal and perfect image. In the anecdotes that we offer at the end of this chapter, some of this will be very clear in our own identification as teachers, and we hope this makes it apparent that we are neither immune to nor outside of the

[1] Notably the Initial Teacher Training Core Content Framework (DfE, 2024), the Teachers' Standards (DfE, 2021), and the Education Inspection Framework (Ofsted, 2023), all structure the daily life of the teacher in the UK, not just at the level of expectation but also in the construction of fantasy. A certain figure of teacher is formed in these policies, a great teacher' (DfE, 2024) at that.

Lacanian critiques we raise. No doubt there exist an array of descriptors, other signifiers, that make a good teacher and indicate what a teacher should be or do. In the pursuit of this book to outline the figure of the Lacanian teacher, the question 'why teach at all?' is undergirded by the structure of fantasy.

Fantasies can come to breed discontent amongst teachers in the impossibility of attaining them, discontent that is not just psychic but material too. As Britzman notes (1991, p. 66), and has been seen in any wave of teacher union strikes in the past few decades, the shared investment in fantasies of teaching foreclose the possibility of fighting for improvements in the material conditions of their workplace. Attempts to do so are quickly reformulated as greed or laziness, as the teacher occupies a mythic position embodying a redemptive fantasy that must be appealing in and of itself. These fantasies are commonplace and quotidian, yet at the same time fabulated and fantastical. They are multiple, and of course often intersecting.

The Lacanian perspective would insist that our ideas of the teacher figure, and our desires in relation to that figure, are necessarily and significantly informed by fantasy. For Freud, 'psychic reality' is predicated on fantasy, that is to be strictly differentiated from illusion. Fantasy is an ever-present energy that informs our conduct, our actions, our disposition and comportment whether consciously or not. Freud drew an analogy with fantasy and the idea of a 'nature reserve' (SE XV, p. 419), a peculiarly modern phenomenon we might say, when so much of the world is dominated by the human presence, with its structures and orderings. For Freud the realm of fantasy—obviously existing alongside what he referred to as the reality principle—was that dimension of the psyche that, like the nature reserve, could exist in a happy state of non-cultivation, allowing its hugely various products to burgeon alongside one another in no particular ordering and with no conscious intervention. In this, for Freud, fantasy is also so much more than mere daydreaming. Fantasy informs psychic life in often dramatic and far-reaching ways, providing a psychically energized dimension to every perception, to identities and to the whole field of human interaction, whether personal and close-up or public and global.

Fantasies are at the level of the ontological in the Lacanian picture. They are not some free-floating, internal property, but rather a necessary aspect of the Imaginary as it shapes our recognition of things out there in the world and contributes to our desires for them. In Lacan's ontological topography that we outlined in Chap. 1, the Imaginary order stands alongside the Real and the Symbolic that both reverberate with its projections. Fantasy is fundamental, feeding desire and interacting powerfully with the drive. That is, how would something be desirable if we did not have fantasy fuelling it? The desire one student holds for a certain university, for example, might be sustained by the fantasy image they have of themselves in that institution, likely laced with images of 'student life' from films and tv and traced with the cache of the signifier of that institution's name. To paraphrase Jacques-Alain Miller (2013), fantasy is the stuff on which desire sustains itself, but only to miss the direction the drive points it towards.

The object desired in fantasy,[2] say a promotion to Head of Department or a more attentive class that will do the assigned reading, situates the subject as determined by it and coordinates the signifier and enjoyment of the subject. The fantasy acts as a montage that fixes enjoyment, shielding the subject from the Real, and as such shares much in common with anxiety relative to its protective function (X, p. 41). Dominant fantasies of teaching will only come to breed anxiety through time in the impossibility of fully embodying them (VIII, p. 363). But anxiety may also operate as a protection interposing itself between the subject and the threat of a traumatic encounter with the Real. In identifying with different figures of teachers, we are protected from encountering an educational Real—the horrifying aspects of it that slip through the teacher's fingers by holding onto our supposed similarity with some salvific or redemptive figure.

The mode of fantasy is also important: it is 'a staging of desire that always includes a subject, defines who they are as divided in their enjoyment and suffering, and objects which they think, at an unconscious level, will bring satisfaction' (Parker & Pavón-Cuéllar, 2021, p. 115). The use of 'staging' in relation to both fantasy and teaching is interesting. Fantasy has a theatrical quality, and we are again making links to the Mirror *Stage* of Lacan's theory of ego destitution. In our imagination or dreams, but also on screen or in speech, we find the image of a subject playing the part of

[2] The structure that Lacan provides is $ <> *a* for both fantasy and anxiety. It indicates a relationship (<>) between the subject ($) and the object cause of desire (*a*). We have already gone into much detail about the teacher as a subject in the previous chapter and outlined objet a there and in the glossary. See also Stock (2024b) for a lengthier account of this matheme in relation to the fantasy of natural education as found in Rousseau, Sade, and contemporary schooling. This relationship or 'lozenge' is what characterises the subject's relation to the object cause of their desire. Its shape posits that they are both more than > and less than < their desire (XI, p. 209), a relationship both backwards and forwards, a 'contrary relationship between the two sides' (Ormrod, 2014, p. 99).

seeking something we think we might want. But teaching itself, as we will make clear in the next chapter and beyond, is also already a sort of staging. The space of the classroom has a fantasmatic quality to it, as the screen or whiteboard that frames the teacher allows them to perform in a frame, as if on a screen or theatre stage (Herbert, 2012; Stock, 2024a). In this way, we see not only the fuel of desire but also 'the inertia which fantasy provides to the desire' (Miller, 2009, p. 1). In teachers' identification with fantasmatic figures, they arrest desire from wanting much else beyond what is available in the fantasy already. They will just play the part, as it were.

What is at stake here, then, is the way we identify with a signifier and all its inherent imaginaries, including the fantasies we see on screen or in education policy. As we said in the previous chapter, the answer to the question 'What am I?' (VIII, p. 240) is an identification with a signifier, is a form of incarnating, cystallizing (p. 240) the ego-ideal, arresting the figure. When one enunciates 'I am a teacher', there is *nachträglichkeit*, retroactivation of the subject's life to be teacherly, now arriving at its terminus or 'endpoint' (p. 241). Everything the subject sees in their past experiences is part of that signifier; but when taking it on, we terminate desire. No longer does one, the subject who has proclaimed themself as a teacher, desire. Now one desires what 'a teacher' desires, and that teacher is fuelled by the world of fantasy out there in the world.

We are aware, as teachers ourselves, how subjected we have been to such fantasies, many that we likely, if at least unconsciously, hold onto, in spite of our claims to have transcended them here. We do not occupy a meta-position that Lacan makes clear is impossible to occupy (III, p. 326). Much of the media cited below are sources of great pleasure to us, despite their shortcomings. Many of the examples given in this chapter and elsewhere are personal, thus we hope that readers will be able to pursue their own fantasmatic formations of teaching as a means of tackling their identification with the subject position of the teacher.

Born to Teach

> No one is born a great teacher. Great teachers continuously improve over time, benefitting from the mentoring of expert colleagues and a structured introduction to the core body of knowledge, skills and behaviours that define great teaching. (DfE, 2019a, p. 3)

This quote from the UK Department for Education's (DfE) reforms of Initial Teacher Training (ITT) sheds some ironic light on the question concerning the image of the teacher. The language of continuity, of becoming, implies the importance of development specific to the being of the educator, envisioned as an ongoing, even interminable progress through a career journey. At the same time, this statement clearly signifies the notion of an achievable terminus. The implicitly ongoing process must be directed towards the grand goal of being the 'great teacher'. Amid the affirmation of becoming, allied to the outlining of key required dimensions ('knowledge, skills and behaviours') we find an implicit end, an ideal state. Despite the negative use of the idiom 'born to teach' by the DfE, it is difficult to claim that this fantasy does not suffuse the being of many teachers, ourselves included. Indeed, we might even state that its negative use in the DfE statement transforms it into *objet a* for the teacher seeking identification with a fantasmatic image.

Contradictory logic aside, the projection of the ideal-ego, set against specific dimensions of being, implies a delimiting of the subject of the teacher. This governmental model of the teacher positions the teacher-to-come as subject to and of the ideal. The official ideal of the teacher figure is given form and shape in certain signifiers, outlined in official documents, that enframe professional assessment and development discourses and practices. In the Lacanian sense, the likes of the DfE exist as part of the already powerfully governing Symbolic order of education, responsible for both delivering but more likely repeating educational fantasies. Though bodies like the DfE and English school inspectorate (Ofsted) are often positioned as antithetical to the goals of teachers (Ellis, 2024), they exist within a governing structure of language that engulfs all teachers. In our exploration of the signifiers the teacher may enunciate in this chapter, it will become clear that this Symbolic order imposes a continuity between these supposedly oppositional bodies of teachers and government. What's more, in moving to other dimensions of the Symbolic order in general educational discourse, we will see how the chain of signification is metonymic, that is, associatively linked, throughout.

Like the DfE, Ofsted as a master signifier of antagonism towards the Symbolic world of the teacher, contribute to the fantasy. The 'Self-Evaluation Form', popular with Ofsted in the past (2015) and on the agenda again with teacher union sponsored organisation Beyond Ofsted (2023) is the central document of inspection. Lesson observations are now often sandwiched with a pre-observation self-evaluation ('how do you think it will go?') and a post-observation self-evaluation ('how do you think it went?'). It assumes and leads the internalization of the ego ideal within the institution of the school as a subject for inspection where the 'views of the children... [and] professionals' (Ofsted, 2015, p.6) are expressed. The performative force of interpellation could not be more emphatic. The point from which the subject now feels the pressure of paranoid scrutiny is located within itself; indeed, it is the notion of a 'within', a core, a self-presence that the Self-Evaluation Form verifies. This core is, of course, meant to be teacherly in some form. The Self-Evaluation Form signifies the very condition of an inner identity, an identity that is nevertheless on show and inspected to ensure that it is true to the ideals that it is ontologically licensed to exist by. Ontology is realized, here, in the gap that is opened as the self through a certain misrecognition of bureaucracy as the signified, when instead it is merely a signifier.

A fantasy we are starting to trace, therefore, is the fantasy of the natural, the one who teaches effortlessly, without thinking, without planning. It is inside them. This teacher, no matter what struggles they face in their personal life, no matter how hard the class is to teach, no matter how tedious the material, will still teach a great lesson and can attest to as much by being to evaluate themselves. As a trainee teacher, one of us recalls being told by a mentor that they should teach a 'doorhandle lesson', the implication being that the whole lesson was planned on entering the classroom. Implicitly, once the teacher as subject enters the space of the classroom, the lesson will simply materialise. This is because one of us believed he was born to teach. The other, as an experienced, confident teacher recalls subscribing to a transposed form of the proud boast of George Solti, then conductor of the Chicago Symphony Orchestra, who related his post-war experiences of conducting on the hoof so that he became so proficient that he 'could conduct the dirt on the wall' ... Now that same teacher, no longer teaching, is haunted by dreams of unplanned lessons, untaught syllabi and lost timetables. Britzman references a similar fantasy she found uttered to her by others:

> The phrasing "teaching in your sleep" is labile enough to invite a teaching phantasy: Wouldn't it be great if we could discover that the secret of teaching is so simple that it can be done with eyes closed? I think that students may believe this about some of their teachers. (2015, p. 133)

We would go a step further and say that some teachers believe this about themselves too. Such images are abundant in the media as an image of méconnaissance (I, p. 167), 'the structures of systematic misrecognition and objectification that characterize ego formation' (E, p. 94) for the teacher. Seeing what we believe ourselves to be on screen, we attempt to embody them in the belief we will be satisfied in inhabiting its image (and of course only feel disappointment and anxiety in its impossibility (VIII, p. 363)). Teachers on screen are predominantly produced in the image of being born to teach: as in *Dead Poets Society, Dangerous Minds, The Ron Clark Story, Freedom Writers,* the list could go on.

Though a useful figure, in moving beyond the oft-cited example of Mr Keating in *Dead Poets Society* (see Clarke 2019 for a Lacanian critique of that film), we turn to some others. The 2006 film *Half-Nelson* begins with history teacher Dan Dunne (played by Ryan Gosling) sitting unshaven in his underpants, staring into the abyss as his alarm clock goes off. We are confronted with the figure of the heartthrob at his lowest ebb, and though the clear intention is to represent what we will soon learn is Dunne's drug addiction, there is an interesting eroticism at play in this half naked figure of the teacher who prepares for his day. Cigarette smoked to the nub, aviator glasses on to hide his eyes, Dunne gets out of his car and walks into his classroom—unsurprisingly a group of predominantly black students in echoes of the white saviour narrative seen so often on the screen (see the next fantasy *Making a Difference*). Dunne rubs his bleary eyes and cranes his neck up at the class in an exhausted movement. But then, the metamorphosis occurs: 'What is history?' he asks the class. The students make jokes, which Dunne responds to with quick wit, then his face, body and voice become animated as if raised from the dead. As he begins to give the class an outline of dialectics and the civil rights movement, certainly not a coincidental topic in such a fantasy, he is reborn, reborn to teach. The class erupts into bouts of humour and outpourings of knowledge, calling out examples of dialectical relations, mocking each other with misogynist jokes, recalling dates of resistance. One student even recognises the power relation at play in the classroom between teacher and student. A great teacher teaches the student about the imbalance between them, after all. *Half Nelson* goes on to chart the descent of Dunne as his drug addiction takes over. We even see an ethical disaster as he buys crack from a student. And yet, the lessons depicted throughout the film remain broadly engaging and compelling, suggesting he can fight through his suffering when teaching is on the cards.

Perhaps a more quotidian, thus a more effective example, exists in the 2000–2004 UK TV series *Teachers*, an honest and comedic portrayal of the British comprehensive education system. Though the show offers a pantheon of images of teachers, ranging from the purely sexualised to the totally incompetent, the English teacher Simon Casey (played by Andrew Lincoln) occupies the central role. Series 1 sees his binge-drinking, disorganisation, and sloppiness somehow materialise into a full-time job at the school (likely a jibe at the state of the British comprehensive school). Nothing compounds this image of his half-arsed attitude more than the same tie he wears in every episode that he pulls out of his locker at the start of the day, fighting a hangover from the previous night. It is halfway through the second series that the fantasy fully materialises whilst Casey is reluctantly covering for Penny Neville, another teacher in the department that everyone believes to be a great teacher. The lesson begins and, like Dunne in *Half Nelson*, the animation of the body and voice occurs. Previously slumped on a sofa in the staff room, now he claps his hands together and writes on the board with intentional verve, shouting 'Shut it!' sarcastically to the class. The clap and gesticulation so commonly seen on screen are the somatic signifier of the great teacher. He sets them a task to keep them occupied, allowing him to sit back in his chair and return to the sedentary figure, only to soon realise that the class know nothing of the text they have supposedly been taught. So it is that he returns to occupy the teaching space, transforming once more into the man born to teach despite all the circumstances that plague him. The lesson ends and a student says 'Cheers Sir, it wasn't too bad!', a thumping complement from the stereotypically disaffected youth of the series.

Mr Casey, so 'down to earth', born to teach, remains just as pervasive and strong now in recruitment adverts for teacher training commissioned by UK's Department for Education. In a predictably named advert *Every Lesson Shapes a Life. Tuesday* (DfE, 2022), a humdrum day of teaching is also punctuated by a disaffected student shouting 'Nice one Sir' at the end of the school day. Indeed, one of us even recalls being in town with their young son one evening and going into McDonalds. They were spotted by a young man who stood in front of the busy 'restaurant' pointed at them and shouted 'Fucking wicked teacher!' They had long ceased to teach in school and had only known the person in question in a disciplinary context. For a moment they felt the eighteen-year teaching stint had been worth it.

The 2020 Danish film *Another Round* [*Druk*] takes a slightly different route to depict the fantasy of the born to teach subject, instead focussing on the cynicism and disaffection of the teacher later into his career. In this overturning, teacher Martin (played by Mads Mikkelsen) has lost his way, finding no pleasure in the space of the classroom. Through turning to Skårderud's theory that the human body has a blood alcohol deficiency easily overcome by a regimented intake of booze, Martin starts to find his place as a teacher again. The drink literally brings him to life, but its potency is most visible in the classroom. More animated scenes materialize of children laughing and shouting out answers as Martin gesticulates around the room. In these examples, we see over and over the transformative movements and voice of the teacher who is innately brilliant, whose command over the class is second nature to him. It is often a 'him', we should note. It is difficult not to identify an aspect of the male fantasy in these depictions, always handsome young men who combine their masculine lasses-faire attitude with their ease of discipline and teaching (Francis, 2008). Anyone who has mentored young male trainee teachers might see their relentless attempts to embody this figure, missing deadlines, skipping lesson plans, arriving late, but of course claiming their students love them. But this fantasy rests on another.

Making a Difference

Another common response that you will hear from would-be teachers when asked why they want to teach is that they want to 'make a difference'. In our own experiences, in mediatised depictions, and in sociological research (Lortie, 1975, p. 28; Schutz et al., 2001, p. 303; Heinz, 2015; Bergey & Ranellucci, 2025), teachers are dominantly envisioned as 'influential agents of change' (Clarke & Kennedy, 2024, p. 2), purveyors of altruistic goods. This dominant fantasy, the reformer, saviour, or redeemer, is of course one that Lacan himself recognised and that we began this book with: 'we place no trust in altruistic feeling, we who lay bare the aggressivity that underlies the activity of the philanthropist, the idealist, the pedagogue, and even the reformer' (E, pp. 80–81). His discussion here is directly related to the misrecognition of the fantasmatic image in his presentation of the mirror stage as recounted in the previous chapter. Such an impulse is not only manifest at the level of the image, but the teacher's discourse too. The belief in 'making a difference' is always loaded with a positive orientation, for of course, 'difference' could be negative, destructive, harmful, and so on. Whenever a teacher cites the fantasy that they want to make a difference, what they might mean is they want to affect a positive change on the students they teach—a positivity that presumes to know the desire of the Other. We have already discussed the ceaseless optimism found in the Symbolic order of education, but clearly this phrase has great importance in teacher's fantasies. Where the Lacanian critique goes further is in recognising not the harmful or even the benign nature of the teacher, but in the unknowability of this impact. As Lacan says, 'nothing we say fails to entail consequences. Yet we don't know which ones' (XVI, p. 23). Every word out of the teacher's mouth is doing something, but it cannot be neatly ordered in the upwards curve of the educational Symbolic. Something always escapes it.

The Ron Clark Story, a televised fictionalisation of the celebrated American educator taking his first job in Harlem, is straightforward in its fantasy of both being born to teach and making a difference. Working against the odds to reach a disaffected and negatively racialised student group, the breakthrough culminates in a scene where the class sit round a birthday cake in party hats and light candles to bluntly symbolise their new beginnings. They turn their back on their path of truancy, crime, anger, and so on, and turn to love learning. There is even the starkly symbolic moment of a student being asked to 'choose a path' between going out to commit robbery or go with his teacher to prepare for the test. Of course, they go on to achieve dizzying test scores, confirming what we have believed all along: that the teacher makes a difference. We are thus demanded to recognise the normative development of the child that *will* occur *if* the teacher's pedagogy is up to the task.

A little more obliquely, the film *Dangerous Minds* presents a narrative where the teacher is represented in dramatic form as the transformative figure, the outsider who is close in sympathy to her charges and who operates with a dedicated ethic of care—something clearly inflected with a feminine figure rather than the masculine ones we have identified thus far. Interestingly, if predictably, this ethic is not rooted in sociological knowledge or socialist principles. It is represented more in the style of a personal attribute, rather like the familiar 'noir' detective's inexplicable commitment to integrity of conduct and the pursuit of truth.

The narrative takes a characteristic and recognizable form with some interesting variations. The teacher-hero LouAnne Johnson (Michelle Pfeiffer) is represented as different from the body of teachers. She is distinguished from the somewhat jaded professional who in effect has given up on the 'academy' kids and distinguished from the administrative bureaucracy which is concerned to maintain procedural proprieties. This difference is in terms of commitment, care, 'charisma' and is expressed in a resourcefulness which goes beyond the limits of given practice. The difference is also the signifier of her clothes. LouAnne Johnson begins to dress casually, reflecting her developing personal-professional style. Her deportment is more varied and informal; she has recourse to a wider range of speech repertoires than colleagues and, interestingly—in terms of a politics of (the representation of) teaching materials—she deploys more 'unconventional' material and terms of reference, bridging with popular culture.

LouAnne Johnson appears as an unlikely, even reluctant entrant, uncertain, untrained but with a romantic view and a commitment 'to teach'. She combines a worldly knowledge with an ability to exert authority and to control by commanding attention, showing us how students will follow when they can sense the difference being made to them by the teacher. Still, she emphasizes the capacity for individual choice: 'There are no victims in this class', but she also fails to save Emilio, for instance. In a neat self-referential irony Emilio reminds 'us', as he reminds his would-be saviour-teacher, that he has 'seen the same movies as you have'. We are implicated in the film at this moment, perhaps emphasising the entanglement with fantasy for the teacher and the student.

There are of course images of teachers who overturn the narrative of the saviour teacher fantasies, though it is telling that they are rarely western cinema and thus escape the dominant educational Imaginary offered by the hegemony of western schooling. *Monsieur Lazhar* begins with a teacher's suicide inside the classroom, a haunting encounter with education's Real. But unlike Mr Clark or LouAnne Johnson who enter a room of racialised Others to save them, substitute teacher Lazhar, an Algerian immigrant who comes to teach an entirely white class in Quebec in the wake of a school tragedy, is the Other who enters the classroom here. Inevitably, we see Lazhar collide with the injunction to uphold the sacred nature of the curriculum in the typical problem raised in educational fantasies. But we should see that Ron Clark, Mr Keating, LouAnne Johnson, Mr Dunne, hover in the margins of the Imaginary still. Lazhar believes his methods—archaic looking to the other teachers—are imperative for the good of the students. As he demands that primary age children read Balzac, we see his devotion to them manifested in the primacy of education, especially in its efforts to heal the wounds of their loss of the deceased teacher.

The aforementioned DfE recruitment advert with its *Every Lesson Shapes a Life* (2022) tagline makes no attempts to mask its depiction of the teacher who makes a difference. The changes seen to the disaffected student who proclaims 'Nice one Sir' at the end are one such example, but more pivotally there are numerous other moments to emphasise the fantasy. Lights are switched on in a darkened classroom at the start of the advert, not only a sign of the teacher's 'early riser' drive to make a difference, but also of the light that will be bestowed on the children in his classroom. Students march up the stairs of the school, at once their ascent to the classroom and towards their futures.

But less banal depictions still retain the trace that teachers are making a difference to the lives of their pupils and to society writ large. The 2011 film *Detachment*, a far bleaker image of teaching, regularly weaves the attempts to improve the lives of children with education's unconscious. Blackboard animations of teachers committing suicide conclude scenes of difficult encounters with parents and students, angry voices on the phone about the viciousness of teenagers are interspersed with the voice of Hitler—the epitome of the Authoritarianism personality that lingers in the voice of teachers (see the section *By Any Means Necessary* below). Students spit at teachers, swear at them, threaten to have them assaulted, and yet, inevitably, as one teacher remarks: 'I don't know what to do with myself when I'm not in the classroom': another 'born teacher', but most importantly one that still retains the imperative to make a difference. Despite *Detachment's* ceaseless reminders of the thankless nature of teaching, the way it hollows one out (Brody identifies as a 'faceless man in an empty classroom' later in the film), by the end it's clear the students will miss him: 'All the other teachers are dickheads'. Brody even goes on to adopt a child prostitute he has been caring for throughout the film, a sign that even if he failed to save the students en masse, at least he saved someone. The impulse to save remains, whilst also constituting the figure of the other than needs saving.

The teacher must be entwined pedagogically with another to impact them. Fantasies of children in educational settings are just as loaded, and in turn give further weight to identification with the signifier of the teacher in the relationship between the two. 'Who needs to be saved?' has dialectical formation on those that save. Though we spend less time on them due to the teacher being the dominant focus of this book, there is much to be found in the Romantic or pastoral construction of the child (Stock, 2024b). One example of such a child needing saving, as in Bibby (2011, pp. 19–20), is the blooming flower that in turn positions the teacher as embodying the nourishment of mother nature (sun, rain), or its failure to provide (storm, drought). The signifiers of food in education create a similar relationship: digestion, chewing on, feeding, and so on (pp. 48–49). Both summon the Freudian figure of the archaic mother popularised by Kristeva (1982) and Creed (1993), and as Bibby says:

> Social fantasies about teachers are multiple but they are very similar to those of the perfect mother: a near telepathic ability to know their learners, super-organisational powers, creative ideas for engaging all children at all times and, above all, boundless love and self-sacrifice. (2011, p. 39)

Both mother nature and the maternal mother as giver of the breast are undoubtedly pervasive in fantasies of the child common in some domains of education as nourishing and caring figures. But it is striking that, with some exceptions, in the more popular Imaginary these maternal signifiers are arguably elided by more phallic, paternal ones—ironic considering the proportion of women in the profession.[3]

The maternal is not fully exorcised from the teacher's Imaginary, however, but rather enfolded into the more dominant masculine one through pastoral logic. In suffusing the teacher's fantasy with both boundless love and paternal knowledge/power, making a difference is further assured. As Copjec states, the 'ideal father' is a 'kinder and gentler' (2015, p. 155) figure, a 'place of knowledge … often imagined under the traits of the educator' (p. 155). Indeed, this combination significantly determines the identity of the teacher figure in modernity. It has a powerful ambiguity in its relation with the disciplinary function and these two dimensions—pastoral/discipline—which may correspond as we said to a stereotypical feminine/masculine divide (one, of course, that depends powerfully on the fantasmic property of the signifier). The impersonal given order of

[3] This irony is of course not accidental. The Symbolic of education, like any institution of modernity, ceaselessly enacts the carving of sexual difference around the phallic function (see Chaps. 4 and 5) that Lacan examines in Seminar XX. In education, we now see a demand for "positive" forms of masculinity in the belief of the teacher as a powerful and influential role model, adding to the fantasy that boys can be saved (and thus girls too) by a good teacher. This has certainly shaped the necessity of male teacher imaginaries being made readily available and even resulted in 'teaching manfully' (Francis, 2008, p. 109)—a masculine bodily embodiment of the dominant teacher fantasy (Vick & Martinez, 2011). Pedagogy, in this sense, becomes gendered by educational fantasms, just like the classic image of Mr Keating standing with his legs apart proudly on his desk.

knowledge stands as a form of big Other against which the two modalities of being can be played out. It is interesting to consider this in relation to the vast social transformation that comes with the installation and development of state education (Hunter, 1994), where education's governmental role operates at the most intimate level producing not just disciplined bodies and hierarchically ordered subjects of knowledge, but that also engage with and manage identities at the psychic level. Consider, in contemporary schooling, the impetus given to the ethical dimension where teachers are adjured to promote qualities of 'character' (DfE, 2019b). The nurturing fantasy is written into the discourse of much intertextual material in schooling, so that, independently of individual gender orientations of teachers, maternal and maieutic metaphors can dominate.

At the same time, these metaphors of provision and nourishment are orally driven, that students should swallow and ingest what they are taught (VIII, pp. 200–202) There is an important breakthrough of the Real to identify here, as what is ingested is only to be evacuated as shit (p. 203). What if we don't make a difference? Britzman makes this clear in her assertion that 'Being forgotten goes against the teacher's fondest wishes, or the idealizations we have been schooled by: that no matter what happens, we teachers are memorable characters for our students no longer' (2015, p. 136). So too does Webster make a similar claim about the end of analysis for the analyst, who is to be 'Flushed away like a piece of shit' (Webster, 2022, p. 81). The inverse of the McDonalds anecdote given earlier is when one of us was walking down a street in town and seeing a student that they believed thought highly of them, only for the student to ignore them and keep walking. Flushed away like shit, they were confronted with Real that the fantasy allows us to ignore.

Subject Specialists

Still a young teacher, one of us applied for a teaching job in 2012. The final lines of the cover letter are as follows:

> *The culmination of my career thus far has shown me the impact a teacher can have on a pupil, and I am proud to be in the position of such influence. I feel my experiences at school bestowed me with the love for English I have today, and indeed many of the staff inspired me to chase the profession. It would be affirming, to say the least, for me to teach and guide activities in such a fostering environment, thus continue the cycle with an independent and zealous group of pupils.*

There is much to analyse (and perhaps to lament) here, but something that is clear in the intersecting discourses of teaching is the passion, even adoration and love they have for 'their' subject. As in Chap. 2, teachers at all levels 'have' a subject that they teach, in the form of a specialism they are expected to enjoy some mastery of so to be able to teach students to the level required. Both writers of this book are Literature 'specialists' who taught English as a subject and we claim Literature teachers stand as the fantasy of the teacher *par excellence* in educational imaginaries. Often the image of the inspiring teacher on screen takes the form of an English teacher working with their students through some great work of literature (beyond the obvious example of Robin Williams' Mr Keating reciting poetry in *Dead Poets Society,* Drew Barrymore's teaching of Graham Greene's *The Destructors* to the alienated and cynical Donnie in *Donnie Darko*; Adrian Brody's teacher in *Detachment* is a brooding English teacher who writes prose; *Teachers* focusses predominantly on an English department; the eponymous *Monsieur Lazhar* teaches Balzac to young children; LouAnne in *Dangerous Minds* wants the troubled class to love Dylan Thomas, via Bob Dylan).

There are regular debates over specialisms in teaching. UK's teaching regulatory body Ofsted criticise some schools for their lack of overt subject specialism in their staff, and indeed a recent Ofsted review of the English curriculum across the entirety of the UK lambasted professionals due to gaps in subject specialism. References to 'foundational knowledge' and 'subject knowledge' of the 'history and development of literature', 'craft of the writer', and 'nature of literary study' (Ofsted, 2022) overtly signify the importance of one specific model of subject specialism for teaching English in the classroom. Similarly, the reforms to the teacher training sector in England (DfE, 2024) generated core standards for teachers on their training programmes to be adapted to subject specifics. This relation between the mastery of a subject and the teacher as a subject is thus upheld as essential to the shaping of the figure who must operate within the world of education outlined in the preface. Subject knowledge is one of many signifiers the teacher must confront to arrive at the point of becoming a teacher. We both recall so-called formative experiences in our English classrooms as students where the teacher at the front of the classroom dazzled us with their encyclopaedic knowledge of literature, fully recounted in the close of this chapter.

The classic English teacher, perhaps embodied in John Dixon's (1967) seminal book, *Growth through English*, carries a special burden. Dixon's collectively achieved new subject model defined the essence of the subject in terms of 'personal growth', so that English wasn't merely a subject on the curriculum and nor merely the locus for encyclopaedic knowledge of literature. It was crucially about sensitivity, about reading the world, about self-expression. One of us recalls at the beginning of his teaching career joining a new and large comprehensive school and being adjured by the avuncular headteacher to remember that as teachers the most important thing that we teach is ourselves. He meant that our conduct and comportment matter to students, but there is also the sense that, as English teachers, in particular, we are engaging with ways of feeling, ways of seeing, knowing and being-in-the-world. The headteacher in question was no Heideggerian, but he put his finger on an important ontological dimension that English teachers at that time, especially, were prone to accede to. Subject identity was being reframed, liberalized and freed from the shackles of an emphasis on canonical literature and standard language. Instead, the dominant fantasy, proposed by Dixon, among others, and endorsed later in the 1974 Bullock Report on the Teaching of English (HMSO), was of the traditional figure of the teacher, close to her students, engaging in mutually enriching extension of their worlds of feeling, knowing and being. Only the English teacher could take on this missionary work that addressed the sensibility as well as the linguistic competence and cultural orientation of their charges.

It is interesting too that such figures as Dixon's English teacher are curiously intellectual, a caché that comes with the signifier certainly of English teacher, if not teacher more broadly for some. Adrian Brody's Mr Barthes in *Detachment* stitches together many of these images. His name, an obvious allusion to Roland Barthes, a significant French intellectual who himself claimed that the teacher and the intellectual often inhabit the same space (1977, p. 190), is coupled with the early shots of writing tortured prosed late into the night, reading novels on the bus, a camera tracking him around night-hawk city walks, cigarettes before class. The surplus enjoyment of this figure rests so clearly in fantasy, and even in, or perhaps especially in, the knowledge of this fantasy. The image of Edward Said in his Harvard Office in his Saville Rowe tweed, holding his Scheaffer pen, or of Jacques Derrida walking down the street with his coat collars turned up and pipe in mouth, is a trope that so many in the academy fantasmatically entertain in the pursuit of enjoyment, something that seeps into some fantasies of teaching too. (One of us spent so long droning on about Said's pen—which has been mentioned a few times in this book—to a class that a student bought it for them as a leaving present). But more interestingly, as is made clear in the Lacanian operations of jouissance, it is through the signifier that this enjoyment occurs. So it is that when I pull out a fountain pen in a meeting (whilst others produce biros) I can subjectivate myself through the signifier as the image of the scholar. One might wonder if this fantasy has started to wane in the profession at little, and perhaps contributed to what we perceived as disillusionment in it when leaving teaching and pursuing academia. But perhaps it still lingers in what teachers lament when they bemoan the state of education—a return to a mythical state of intellectualism, sophistication, and subject passion.

By Any Means Necessary

In Damian Chazelle's 2014 film *Whiplash,* J.K. Simmons' Fletcher, a violent jazz orchestra conductor and teacher, tortures his students, particularly Andrew Neiman, to push them to playing at an unthinkable level. The drum in the film occupies the position of *objet a* in its perfect form, an object with a rim-like structure that can never be wholly accessed, only grasped towards and beaten around the edges (XI, p. 168). The pressure and intensity of the drive are thrashed into the skin of the snare, producing the sound that initiates the film. At the beginning of the film we hear the sound of the snare as Andrew Neiman practises relentlessly in a darkened room; a mysterious figure appears silhouetted at the door. This formless shape, a space that will soon be inhabited by Fletcher, bursts into the room and demands the drive be mastered. 'Show me your rudiments,' he, the Other, demands. 'Double time swing.' Neiman obeys, and so begins the torment he will undergo throughout the film to exercise his mastery over the drum. The drum in the classroom can be any old bit of content, like a text, a term, a way of thinking, an essay style, a theory, and so on.

As a conductor of a jazz orchestra, Fletcher represents an interesting form of the teacher fantasy, one that seems to occupy the space of the elusive big Other. Fletcher has perfect control as he flicks his wrist and the band launch into their performance. Not only does he command the band, but he owns the music symbolically. As Neiman mangles the beat again and again, Fletcher repeats it is 'Not quite my tempo' (though we soon suspect that there was nothing wrong with Neiman's tempo, and only that Fletcher wishes to torture him). This totalised control of the Symbolic space of the rehearsal room has resonance with the Lacanian figure of the big Other. A fantasm in itself, the big Other is the possessor of the Symbolic. They hold all the signifiers, and as such, must vindicate our use of them. Of course, this figure cannot exist any more than Fletcher does, but it is an essential concept for the possibility of the enunciating subject for Lacan, just as the figure of Fletcher as in total possession of the space and tempo in *Whiplash* is essential for the logic of the film and the fantasy of the teacher. Previously we recounted the passionate and loving teacher as a master of their subject, something there are traces of here as well. So too does this big Other-like teacher have total control of not just the knowledge at play but also of the subjects within the order. Neiman, after getting the tempo wrong once again, has a chair thrown at his head by Fletcher. A clear image of castration by the Other, it is something he must accept in his 'path' (as he calls it when he dumps his girlfriend) to mastery of the drum. Amusingly, the chair throw is a repetition of the fantasy of Charlie Parker's subjectivation as a jazz great—an anecdote shared at the start of the film where Parker has a cymbal thrown at his head.

Fletcher is fired for his conduct. But he makes his method clear:

> I don't think people understood what it was I was doing at Shaffer. I wasn't there to conduct. Any fucking moron can wave his arms and keep people in tempo. I was there to push people beyond what's expected of them. I believe that is … an absolute necessity. Otherwise, we're depriving the world of the next Louis Armstrong. The next Charlie Parker.

If the previous fantasies are retained, making a difference, being a born teacher, being an intellectual, what we might find is a figure like Fletcher is the predictable stitching together of them, the 'join' (X, p. 172) as Lacan has it. Fletcher believes, and perhaps many of us teachers do, that when we are really good in the classroom, we produce the sublime. But this film goes further. It is clear that Fletcher *enjoys* tormenting his students, and perhaps even that the students enjoy exposure to their tormenting teacher in the pursuit of mastery.

Such fantasies, a dialectic of sadism and masochism, are not new to teaching. The French libertine and pornographic philosopher Marquis de Sade was a figure of great interest to Lacan, especially in his essay *Kant with Sade* (E, p. 645). It turns out Sade may be of more importance to educational thinking than he is given credit for (Stock, 2024b). Sade's works are 'relentlessly, tediously educational, perhaps unrivalled in their singular commitment to the course of instruction' (Allen, 2016, p. 41). Quite so: 'Sade has a lot to say about education, challenging in many ways the work of Rousseau that used education as a way to put off corruption from society, cultivate freedom' (Greteman, 2015, p. 612) and so forth.

In the pedagogy of his 1795 educational treatise *Philosophy in the Boudoir*, Sade depicts the teaching of the virginal Eugénie in libertinism through a series of lectures and sexually violent 'activities'. Her tutor Dolmancé, a typical embodiment of the Sadean libertine and of the sadistic teacher, makes great claims throughout about her education as a necessity. Of course, this sadistic act of teaching is to propagate the fantasy that children must learn by any means necessary. Like Fletcher in *Whiplash,* it is acceptable to berate your students and shout abuse at them (something we see in other brutal-pedagogical figures like Dr. Gregory House, or even the dance teacher Abbie Lee Miller on the popular TV show *Dance Moms*), to be violent and throw chairs, to make them learn, read, write, and so on, until their hands bleed. It is acceptable, because it is the duty of the educator. As Žižek neatly encapsulates:

> …the excuse to do our duty should be rejected as hypocritical; suffice it to recall the proverbial example of a severe sadistic teacher who subjects his pupils to merciless discipline and torture. Of course, his excuse to himself (and to others) is: "I myself find it hard to exert such pressure on the poor kids, but what can I do—it's my duty!" (Žižek, 1998 n.p.)

If education occupies, at it seems to in contemporary world culture, an ontotheological primacy, we can see how the figure of the teacher may, at the level of fantasy, take on a masochistic/sadistic character possibility. This may include the self-flagellating teacher, working late into the night, competing with colleagues for the most excessive workload and work ethic, insisting in class that students acknowledge their dedication. This same teacher may exert fearsome discipline, brooking no lapses in concentration, no failures to submit homework. All this frenetic commitment may be justified in relation to a 'necessary' submission to (the big Other) the educational project that is tied not only to self-improvement, but is also essential to the salvation of the world. In this difficult-to-sustain fantasy, the mundane world of the classroom is transfigured.

The Fantasies Enacted

We are now in a position to provide a more thorough account of the teacher and their classroom relations. Having laid out the threads of the teacher in the previous three chapters—ontology, subject, fantasy, we are able to tie them together in their knot. As we have said before, in the field of education, and in relation to discourses concerning teaching and the figure of the teacher, the Lacanian perspective is not commonplace. For the most part, philosophy of education has eschewed the kind of fundamental issues a Lacanian perspective might arouse, taking for granted an already given logic of identities and relations within the educational world order. This foreclosure of questions concerning the most basic phenomenology[4] of education is not accidental. It corresponds with the Lacanian complex of ideas involving the symbolic order, ego-ideal and ideal ego conceived of at the collective level, among others, implicating what we take to be Lacanian ontology (as in Chap. 1). The value of engaging with the Lacanian perspective lies in its ability to disturb what gets taken to be foundational in the order of things, at the ontic level (related to the being of our Being) and, especially, at the phenomenological level where the complexities of subject perception and ideation get activated.

Already, within this ontological configuration of RSI, the figure of the teacher is immersed in 'Borromean' complexity of relations between imaginary projections, ideal representations, and actual social relations within an already complex and overdetermined setting that cannot be broken (XXIII, p. 25). Further, the elements in this configuration indicate already that the field of being is fraught with relational torsions. Our analytic description might sound cool and academic, but our 'being there' is experienced as utterly shot through with desire, drive and is always already

[4] As phenomenology engages with fundamental questions and issues arising from fundamental relations between subjects and objects, including, of course, objects that may be subjects, it seems apt to propose the possibility of a Lacanian phenomenology of the fundamental educational space. This would need to take into account the dynamics of subject relations, subject object relations and the specific properties of educational contexts and their contexts or worlds. If we provisionally refer to this exercise as a phenomenology of the teacher, it is always on the understanding that the teacher is embedded in a specific world, that is also embedded in a larger world. These worldly relations are productive in terms of elaborating the relations between the local, the national and the global, for instance. Phenomenology is fundamental to any philosophy attempting to offer an account of the world, beginning as it does with apparently humble matters such as simple one to one, everyday encounters between subjects and objects … in doing so, in addressing the apparently most basic and most ordinary, phenomenology returns thinking to an essential level and proves that the apparently simple everyday stuff of our encounters with the world are rich in implication and inevitably touch on some far-reaching dimensions of our being. Lacan's thinking clearly touches more than lightly on dimensions of being such as ontology, ethics and epistemology: making Lacan not just an important figure contributing towards modern and contemporary philosophy, but one that challenges some of the fundamental assumptions concerning the very status and integrity of the most basic components of metaphysics including those very subjects, objects and worlds.

at one remove from the Real that will nevertheless break through to trouble the complacency of our conscious individual and collective understandings.

In the first place, we might say, the 'desire of the Other' (MT, p. 38) looms large in the educational settings. Whatever the aspiration or idealization of the individual subject, the teacher is caught in a trap from the outset, a 'rat in the maze' (XX) at the very phase of formation, subjected to statutorily sanctioned scrutiny in terms of performance but also in terms of the acquisition—or adoption—of proper identity, including inspection of appropriate ideation, affiliation and self-projection. The agency of the teacher, a very common signifier in the aim to improve the world of teachers (Priestley et al., 2013, 2015), is always already determined by a series of signifiers—concerning classroom management, adherence to collective institutional values and comportments, delivery of the set curriculum, modes of pedagogy, submission to the educational hierarchy as well as more nebulous categories of being-in-the-world, such as comportment. This daunting array of significations is overseen, as it were, by the master signifier of education that promotes the almost universally adopted educational ethic that populates the world and its 'educational archipelago' (Peim, 2024, p. 139). What's more these signifiers of the being of the teacher are dynamically caught up in the mundane world of practice as well as active in the rhetorics of meaning that beset education at all levels.

The teaching candidate gets confronted by the inevitable interview question. They usually come well prepared, steeped in the significations of educational desire. 'Why do you want to be a teacher?' probes the candidate's desire, anticipating a series of set responses that rarely fail to materialize. The clichéd answers, as we've seen, include reference to 'making a difference', 'changing people's lives', contributing to 'social justice', along with assertions of the 'love' of subject, the desire to communicate that love and thereby to enhance the very quality of others' lives, just as their own has been enhanced by education—all potential examples of the desire of the Other (MT, p. 38) speaking through the teacher. Numerous pieces of research indicate the same sorts of desires (Lortie, 1975, p. 28; Britzman, 1991; Schutz et al., 2001, p. 303; Gorard et al., 2023))—though rarely employ a psychoanalytically informed stance towards the answers provided. Candidate teacher statements are replete with such paeans to education and to both its inward and its external transformative power. Reading through stacks of them gathered through years of accumulation, one is tempted to suspect a secret script that gets passed round. You must enunciate these things to be included into this domain.

In almost all cases, including those where the path to educational enlightenment may not have been without trauma, teacher candidates assert their will to transform, to be the very agents of transformation that can bring about salvation, even if for the very few ready to receive the auratic and mythically imbued 'gift'. Indeed it is interesting how the likes of Lortie (1975), Britzman (1991) and others encounter would-be teachers citing poor experiences of school during childhood, now driven to correct what they did not receive. The very being of the teacher in our time sometimes seems to be predicated on this salvific theme, including the idea of self-salvation, as expressed in the TV adverts analysed above designed to persuade that teaching is imbued with the meaning of life. In saving the saveable, the teacher also saves their own life from the implicit desert of unmeaning beyond the educational realm.

In the training process, now heavily regulated and specified with attainment targets, benchmarks and competences (DfE, 2021, 2024), the teacher candidate is subjected to an ordered judgemental gaze that invites them to see themselves as subject in formation. Teacher educators are subjected to surveillance through observations that judge not only their classroom competencies but that also examine their 'attitudes', ensuring that they share institutional values at local level and beyond. Even matters such as bodily deportment may be subject to an analysis that seeks to alert the trainee teacher to the appropriate choreography of classroom being. The big Other is represented in the figure of the teacher educator, usually a benign, encouraging presence, but one whose being, nonetheless, embodies and expresses the demand of the big Other to engage with the signification order of the dominant teaching ethic. Critique is essential here. One must learn to be evaluative, critical of one's own performance in the name of the ethic of never-ending improvement that education lives by. Matters of classroom control, appropriate differentiation of curriculum delivery, pacing of learning, working towards specified outcomes and so on are all under scrutiny in the light of this remorseless ethical demand.[5]

[5] The figure of the teacher remains caught in this network of scrutiny (including, of course, the self-scrutiny of the superego) that is laden with expectations. The being of the teacher in the educational setting gets significantly defined and projected according to the often-contradictory logic of ideal-ego and ego-ideal. As teacher I must negotiate this difference between how, ideally, I would like to see myself and how I perceive that the authoritative Other ideally wants me to be.

The varied demands of the institution are in turn defined by a specific spatial articulation—classroom, hall, playground in the classic school setting (Peim, 2022; Stock, 2024a)—that represent dimensions of the work of education that the teacher is required sustain: the close-up teacher and learning encounter, the engagement with collective values, the understanding of the meeting of cultures and orientations to meaning. This radical difference in orientations to meaning touches on the huge implications of modes of signification on the effects of teaching, a difference that always disturbs the classical descriptions of pedagogy. This is essential to any Lacanian account of teaching:

> Now, it seems more and more clear to us that this subject who speaks is beyond the ego … It's also the question … to what extent does the symbolic relation, the relation of language, retain its value beyond the subject, in as much as it may be characterized as centred in an ego—by an ego, for an alter-ego? (II, pp. 175–177)

Classroom relations are fraught with differences in relation to the provenance of the signifier, so that what is happening within in the pedagogic scene cannot be accounted for solely in terms of a narrative of teaching and learning, where teaching (the attempted management of the signifier) takes priority for learning, where teaching is deemed to be the cause of learning in a linear logic. The topology of the classroom, no matter how well ordered, how well planned and paced the lesson, how relevant and fascinating the material, is beset by the feedback of the ego whether that be visible or otherwise. The more successful the teacher in the role as pastoral disciplinarian, as supervisor of the signifier, the less visible may be this dimension of otherness, necessitated by the very fact of difference determined by the positionalities of the symbolically ordered scene. But it remains in play, nevertheless, introducing a zone[6] of uncertainty into the logic of the pedagogic scene. This zone takes uncertainty to another level, engaging the shadow realm of desire and the play of the signifier.

[6] This 'zone' is not the ZPD ('zone of proximal development') beloved of the Vygotskians that will be populated soon enough by the ('scientific') signifiers of knowledge proper—now a pop signifier in teacher's professional development too. Indeed, Lacan seems to subscribe to such a zone in his claim that the 'whole point of schooling lies in … anticipating what one may call the child's mental capacities with problems that lie just slightly beyond them' (X, p. 258). But he may of course be saying this ironically, or be demanding that this zone be understood as an 'opening' (p. 258), not as a directing, curing, or bettering.

While we will claim that this logic of uncertainty prevails whatever the context of teaching, clearly there must be significant variables in different settings, for all sorts of reasons, including the level of the discourse, the mode of knowledge in question, and the constitution of the participants. Always framing the pedagogic scene is the world it belongs to, its institutional identity, that may shift its symbolic orientation and redefine something of the relations between participants. Whatever the world, or context, that the pedagogic scene inhabits, it is necessarily structured by the mobile relations between subjects and the symbolic order, their animation by the Imaginary and their constraint by the real. The Lacanian Real is what is beyond the purchase of knowledge or 'symbolization' (E, p. 324). While we may seek to highlight the psychodynamic element in play in educational encounters, the manifestation of the Real is experienced as a permanent possible disturbance in the subject's equanimity; it is always 'in its place' (E, p. 17). The subject doesn't, on this Lacanian view, stand in a cool, detached, contemplative mode before the object or objects of its world. It is always already invested at the level of ideas as expressed in the Symbolic order that seeks to make sense of and categorize the Real. In addition, the subject is beset by the operations of the unconscious, the order of being that operates through metaphor and metonymy to animate the world and its objects above and beyond the conscious management and control of the conscious subject and its accommodation with the symbolic order.

The school, the classroom, the corridor, that staffroom—all the mundane objects in their mundane settings that constitute the world of the teacher—are fraught with these other dimensions and modes that disturb the putative purposes, rationales and modes of being for the teacher. But it would be churlish for us to command an outside of this being. We were taught, teach, are teachers too. We finish by recognising that we too are caught up in these relations by offering our own accounts of "becoming" a teacher, both examples of fantasmatically informed desires that repeat the ones we have explored in the broader Imaginary of education.

For the Rain It Raineth Everyday

It can be difficult to pinpoint the moment one started the journey in becoming something, and of course even when one does it is a product of retroactive fantasy. But this is not always the case with teachers. Often, as with me, there was *a teacher* that the fantasy has been constructed around.

I had four teachers over my two years of studying English A-Level, one of which I consciously acknowledge to be the key inspiration in my becoming an English teacher, and another I partially have to thank for introducing me to postmodern theory (leading to an interest in Derrida that became an interest in Lacan…). But the one who I shall call Mr Rounds gave the lesson that was the primal scene of my teaching.

This was already an era of examination, where results were the only game in town, and the curriculum ruled all. There was little freedom for teachers to 'teach what they wanted to teach', though of course people did and still do find ways. Mr Rounds loved Shakespeare. We-English teachers always talk about the passion for the subject necessary to teach it and bang the drum of 'subject knowledge' when asked about important skills, and Mr Rounds fit that bill. He neglected other parts of the course so to spend longer on Shakespeare (I am certain we studied Ford's *'Tis Pity She's a Whore* but recall absolutely nothing of it). He held a passion for the intellectual life. We read *King Lear* and *Twelfth Night,* both I still count as among the greatest works. Mr Rounds could spontaneously expound the intricacies of the language and form, drawing threads between Elizabethan contexts and modern performances, and I would keenly listen to it all (despite being arrogant, defensive, and uncooperative in all other lessons, including with other English teachers). It was during this time that my romanticisation of Shakespeare began, previously having no strong feelings about him one way or another. It was in a singular moment that this is crystallised by the work of my memory—how funny it is that it does that to us—to form the primal scene of my teaching. The conclusion of *Twelfth Night* is a curious sort of melancholy for a 'comedy', particularly in the words of the fool Feste and his song *When that I was and a little tiny boy.*

I distinctly recall feeling a brush up against my desire when he read this poem aloud (or how I wanted to be seen to be desiring): *For the rain it raineth every day*, says Feste in the refrain. I had found the fools to be the most compelling part of Shakespeare in Mr Rounds' teaching, and here it was that Feste embodied all their wit and insight in one short song (I would regularly teach lessons about Shakespearean fools throughout my career, even in their absence in plays like *The Tempest* or *The Merchant of Venice*). My disaffected affectation, usually so dismissive of anything, was chewed up by the words of Feste, a poignant and melancholic refrain that reminded us of the negativity of Being, coupled with the meta-theatrical distancing and impetus to go on. Perhaps more bluntly, the desire to be seen as an intellectual wrapped itself around the fool's words, an adherence to the idea, to paraphrase Cioran, that only melancholy allows thought to blossom. The 'signifiery' nature of the classroom is so lucid here, how some words from a play could mean so much in my Imaginary identification with them that I would need to go on and make others identify with them too.

By the time I got to university, it was clear to me that I was going to be an English teacher like Mr Rounds, desperate to repeat what I had experienced in that moment (or at least in the condensation of moments and retroactive effects of the primal scene I recalled). I had cemented my identification to another, a figure that I could externally see myself being seen as. I held onto a fantasy of being a writer, too, and wrote fiction often—something else that Mr Rounds had mentioned doing in his own youth. As he told the class that he had written poetry as a teen, the act of a fool no doubt, the class fell silent … shortly followed by a student throwing a book at him in protest at this tragicomic confession. He shrugged and accepted the reaction. I took many creative writing modules at university, and there is another story that could be told about the eventual death (or re-cathecting) of that desire. Still, it is curious how similar scenes to Mr Rounds' fool are at greater work in my memory than ones associated with writing or reading other texts I loved. First coming to love poetry when reading Keats' 'To Autumn', then Eliot's 'Prufrock'. First encountering Joyce's *Portrait,* which I read in one sitting the night before an exam cementing Joyce as the greatest author of all time to me. Then it was Baudrillard as a critical lens for analysing literature. All of these have their own scenes that I could recount—an American postgraduate teaching assistant who always chewed gum and worked as a bouncer and taught me short prose writing; a poetry scholar who had written a poem about The Smiths which adorned her office wall, a lecture on Marlowe that finished with a theatrical rendition of 'Ah, Mephistopheles!' Others too, all of which I had invested some sort of identification or Symbolic grandeur in. But it is funny how now I work through these memories there are many teachers who I idolised and attempted to emulate in some respect, but never think of them like Mr Rounds. He has been manipulated into a stable and unwavering signifier of 'teacher' that I continue to defer to.

I started training to be a teacher immediately after graduating. I was 21 years old, not much older than the A-Level students I would soon be teaching. I knew little literature, being young and having ditched many of my classes at university. I knew even less about language, it not being a feature on my course. In many ways, my 'English education' came through being a teacher, where I would studiously prepare texts and methods for my students and became quite adept at it in the end (my subject knowledge was consistently praised throughout the majority of my career, ironically). My teacher training consisted of placements in two schools, a small, all-girls, inner-city school that made quite an impression on me (I would go on to teach at a similar school for the next six years), and a mixed comprehensive with "challenging behaviour", of which I remember almost nothing. I do recall finding teacher training quite easy and feeling well supported by my politically literate mentor (but would struggle deeply in my first year as a full-time teacher). I gelled with my classes, picked up the texts and the pedagogies quickly, and got on with my departments. I remember feeling important in some way. The first imaginary identification of the subject who makes a difference started to swell, and I found the job even more enjoyable than I thought I might. Living with two friends who had pursued different careers, I found the pile of marking I would bring home a sign of my significance; I had chosen to do something that helped others, the pile said. Perhaps, also, something about thirty children listening to me talking about a Baudelaire poem must have seemed to me like a moment where I was stepping the same steps as Mr Rounds. I would feel this wave of *nachträglichkeit* many times over the next thirteen years of my time as an English teacher, especially when I taught Shakespearean fools.

I also remember feeling upset during my training when I first shouted at a child, something I had promised myself I would not do. This feeling quickly disappeared when I started my first job and many teachers around me seemed to take delight in screaming at children and scaring them. They would have mantras like 'no smiles till Christmas' and some would gleefully share anecdotes about making children cry. I imitated this for a little while too, once again seeking identification with those around me. I was a teacher of Michael Gove's 2014 GCSE reforms, the much-decried reduction of the English curriculum with its supposed focus on rigour. The impetus on exam results only increased, and I would pride myself on being able to navigate both this demand and my desire to continue the sharing of the love of literature I remember experiencing with Mr Rounds. Eventually I went back disliking shouting or the deliberate cruelty so common to some teachers. In my final year of teaching a student asked me why I never shouted at the class (though I did still on occasion). "What difference does it make?" I asked.

Funnily, it was a prerequisite of my teacher training that I should do a week's work experience in a school before applying. I went back to my old school and, naturally, shadowed Mr Rounds for a week. I don't remember how I felt watching him then.

My Father's Birthday

For me, it wasn't until I was almost eighteen that I decided English was my subject, at the moment when I felt that the affiliation, the commitment, the desire was not at all a matter of choice. I felt that I was marked out for English. English had called me and the call was caught up with some of my most intimate connections. I remembered my mother's tattered but elegant copy of Wordsworth poems, its dark blue hard cover, its neat, extensive annotations made in her convent school days. So, it seemed fitting I should study Wordsworth (avidly) at A level. What's more poetry had been important in forging adolescent associations. Some of my friends and my sister's friends had formed a kind of legal samizdat, circulating informal copies of poems we'd written, to be commented on and collected.

I was impelled to read, driven by a powerful series, I think, of interlocking fantasies and a strong sense of a certain portion of the Symbolic order that would reflect an advanced self back to me, a self that could engage in higher level insight and experience. The signifier 'English' alluded to a chain of seductive signifiers, carrying a serial aura caught up with fantasies of personal, intellectual, cultural distinction, and with fantasies of the possibility of aspiring to a wholeness of being, as well as a certain mastery, not only of literature, but necessarily of 'Life': imagine if you could say you had read George Eliot, Henry James, Dickens, Joyce, T.S. Eliot, Turgenev, Tolstoy; but imagine also if you could silently feel that you had become inward with these figures, these signifiers of distinction, insight, initiated into a very special and exclusive world, attuned to meaning itself and to the highest possible understanding of life, just like the Knausgaard anecdote from the previous chapter. Literature was a portal and subject English was its ground, although one that would make heavy demands if one was to enter its most hallowed places.

There were moments, temporal 'points de capiton' that sealed my subject interpellation, both very intimate and institutionally situated, points or moments when emerging sensations, feelings of attachment or longing got clinched into something more persistent and invasive. I did a Special Paper in English at A level, and my teacher, a powerful if slightly distant figure handed me a copy of T.S. Eliot's *The Waste Land*. Sitting in classes as the teacher offered an informed and informing reading was a bonding experience, not always comfortable as the teacher, in the role of analyst, asked awkward questions that could throw the aspiring ego into fragile uncertainty. Silences were pregnant with the threat of failure, exclusion, incomprehension. The painstaking close reading of this hallowed text, *The Waste Land*, was analogous to an initiation rite, like a reading of an arcane catechism that, if we could endure it meaningfully, offered a thrill of access not like any other. English was clearly a subject that could not be acquired through application, like any other, but demanded that one's very self be put on the line, one's 'sensibility' being at stake.

But then a lesson would explicate some exemplary textual insights. In one General Studies lesson that same teacher read extracts concerning the horse in literature: the dream sequence in *Crime and Punishment*, Vronksy's horse-race in *Anna Karenina*; the opening sequence of *Hard Times*; Yeats's 'The Fascination of What's Difficult'. All of this material was not on any syllabus: but it spoke to a certain longing. It belonged to no determinate field of knowledge, but suggested a liminal world of knowledge that would engage the self, that would exceed mere syllabus knowledge. Something of this 'otherness' was expressed in perhaps unexpected ways: in the style of certain book covers, in the gesture of ambiguity deployed by my English teacher, in the tone of discussions among inductees, in certain quotable phrases. And there were plenty of signifiers to embody the possibility for another kind of access to a certain fulness of being and knowing: F.R. Leavis at that time was the living embodiment of that condition. Leavis affirmed that subject English (always superior to philosophy) was central to any thinking that might challenge the hegemony of 'technologico-Benthamism', that might allow one to navigate the depredations of modernity and ultimately save what was worth saving in our common collective cultural heritage. At the same time, a certain juridical order, the system of public credentials, made its own oppressive demands, experienced as an unnecessary bar to subject fulfilment. The symbolic order of English was fractured into different dimensions, and there was always a price to pay in terms of submission to the relatively mundane demands to gain access to its more elevated peaks. Always the possibility of a certain jouissance, a painful pleasure in the reading of an obscure, uninterpretable text, even while the very reading of it constituted its own accomplishment and held out the possibility of insight and further entry into the hallowed discourse.

It was my father's birthday, 13th December 1971, and we had wine at home to celebrate, an unusual embellishment to evening dinner taken on our knees habitually in front of the television. My teacher called unexpectedly to our upstairs flat in London and my mother answered, downstairs. He had come to announce that I had won a scholarship to Cambridge to read English. I was delighted, having been through the exam and interview process. He invited me to join himself and colleagues for a celebration drink elsewhere. I went and still feel a touch of shame for abandoning my father on his birthday to go off with my new spiritual, intellectual 'father' … I look back on that period of my life as a more or less wilful abandonment of one world, the world of home, of childhood friends for another: the big world of the spiritual and intellectual quest for meaning, where meaning took the specific form of the substance of the subject order accessible through immersion in literature.

Long before university though came the ceaseless work of deciding what was 'proper' to literature and what didn't make the grade. A certain submission to a hieratic, informally regulated content and structure. This became available only through the reading of the cynosures of the subject, the archons of what was judged to be proper to its most serious and most pressing elements. I decided at A level that once the exams were done with I would have to read F.R. Leavis and what was known as 'the Scrutineers' (a group of Leavis apostles who occupied positions of influence within subject identity.)

Becoming a teacher involves new forms of submission, to a newly encountered Symbolic order with its own specific forms of Imaginary and its own forms of demand. Once again, one is thrust into the position of the initiate, impelled to learn the rules of game and to internalize its favoured modes of conduct, its established models and modes of deportment. I entered the profession in 1975 at a time when there was still a flush of excitement about the new order of comprehensive education, initiated by circular 10/65 and reinforced by the 1976 Education Act. There was the sense of a new educational world order in the air and that feeling of a quiet revolution in the name of equality and social justice permeated the very loosely organized PGCE that I underwent. During that year I became interested in the idea of comprehensive education and saw myself committed to its (admittedly vaguely formulated) ideals. I found an English department in a new London overspill comprehensive school that was committed to a left-Leavisite ethic. I was pleased to be part of a vanguard that was determined to bring real literature to the masses, as it were. We taught the subject in conditions of unprecedented and now long terminated freedom, inventing our own syllabuses at all levels. I learned, under the tutelage of Alastair West, my head of department, that it was possible to read Camus with year ten 'mixed-ability' classes, that the 'ersatz English' of accessible literature was not necessary and that Turgenev could be read, enjoyed and made sense of by all. As a department we prided ourselves on our challenging literature choices. CSE candidates could write thoughtfully about Eliot's 'Marina' or Wordsworth's 'Westminster Bridge'. Classes would listen, with sufficient training and the imposition of appropriate discipline, to readings of novels and poems that were conventionally deemed beyond their ken.

For me, this seemed an apotheosis of my teaching career: as an English graduate from an elite university I was privileged to occupy the position of the 'one who knows' to belong to a hieratically distinct class of being, engaged in endless missionary work, able to indulge fantasies of cultural salvation, as a literature guru, bringer of the gift of poetry to relatively culturally impoverished lives. The theological dimension of this nebulous fantasy are obvious, but were always overshadowed by the institutional demand for assessment: the intrusion of the Real in the form of lists of names of candidates submitted for public examination that had to be put into rank order. This disturbing presence, indicative of a fundamental flaw staining the social justice dimension of the educational fantasy, still haunts.

There was, however, a new possibility for the educational fantasy on the horizon. In my 'career' an historical accident in the shape of 11–18 reorganization meant that I felt impelled to seek a position elsewhere and took up a post in Leicestershire, then regarded as the home of progressive state sponsored education. As head of English drama and media in a 14–19 'Community College' in an era of immense curriculum freedom in English (ironically under the Thatcherite Keith Joseph) I was able to promote a vision of the subject with colleagues I had a hand in appointing. At the same time (1983) I received a pre-publication copy of Terry Eagleton's *Literary Theory: An Introduction* that posed a serious challenge to the Leavisite model of subject identity I had been addicted to. In addition, a close colleague had been given a two-year secondment to study at Oxford and was relaying copies of works by Althusser and Bourdieu to me that insisted that the dark shadow of assessment rooted in social class inequality couldn't be suspended in the name of the cultural gift. More positively, it seemed, entirely new and very challenging discourses entered the field of knowledge, often inspired by powerful trends in continental philosophy, linguistics and sociology. New ideas about language, culture and value came into play: the very stuff of English and English teaching. Gradually, it seemed, a new form of subject identity and a series of new (at least to me) fantasies of teaching could be sustained as a new vanguard formed and engaged with meaningful struggle with the old order. The times they were a changing, although not perhaps as I and a handful of others thought. A shift in the order of the clerisy appeared to be in progress. The dominant fantasy that I worked within was the distant but still powerful idea of a long-term transformation—a long revolution, as Raymond Williams had put it—that would restore subject English to its properly demotic function. In the meantime, there was plenty to do in terms of applying those new ways of thinking about language and text in the English classroom under the aegis of the very liberal curriculum arrangements (that were at least partly an inheritance of the Bullock Report).

All of this personal history was of course embedded in a signifying history, where the signifier played the crucial role of enabling the meaning of the fantasy to wait, as it were, in suspended animation, always deferred, but always at the same time in the offing. There were various positions one could take within English teaching, within academic English, within education: and these were organized around their own 'points de capiton', having their own powerfully anchoring signifiers to direct the 'truth' of one's subject being. In my case the key signifiers shifted, interfered with in their substance by ideas, perceptions, readings caught in the intertextual web of conscious engagement, all the while being powerfully bolstered by less conscious agendas such as mastery, redemption, justice—all loaded with meaning that might render the Real of education with its shabby buildings, ambiguously engaged students, internecine staff relations, endless marking and the remorseless grind of the timetable habitable. And of course, even now, as I write this, I will not have shaken off the dimension of fantasy to confront the cold hard reality of the way things actually are in themselves. Retrospective meaning-making restores significance to the narrative of one's fragmented and temporally disjointed life. There are elements of the would-be hero still lurking in the desire to represent oneself—perhaps, as in my case, through the signifiers Derrida, Foucault, Malabou, Freud, Lacan among others—as the one who really knows. And while I acknowledge this dimension of this 'work', I can't quite relinquish the assumed access to the special mode of being-in-the-world afforded by those attachments that are not entirely dissimilar in psychic quality to my teenage attachments to Hemingway, Dostoyevsky, Turgenev, Tolstoy and Eliot, for example.

Traversing Our Fantasies

Reading these histories in relation to Lacan, there arises a constant tension in this affiliation to the subject and one's subject identity, one that is never resolvable through an achieved equilibrium or settlement. Rather like the desire for a loved object, there are traumatic encounters that suggest the essence (or quintessence of the subject other) lies beyond our grasp. We might add that the element of trauma is not episodic, either, that we are, as subject's subjects to some degree traumatised in our subjection and subjectivity. We may have read Turgenev, but what about Lermontov? Pushkin? And what about that exam? We may have achieved 44 out of 50 in a poetry practical criticism exercise, but there remains a six-mark gap, and besides, that was at A level, not at degree level. From a position of incompleteness of possession we constantly stand in a position of wondering what is demanded of us. This torsion in the register of demand occasions a kind of splitting within the ego that seeks identification, recognition and acceptance in the embrace of the subject other. On one hand, I must see myself from the position of the subject as the subject sees me (and judges me to be lacking); on the other hand I may imagine myself as I would want to be seen. There are two of me, at least, in this splitting at the level of the ego as the two points of identification—the ego-ideal and the ideal-ego—conflict with one another. While the conflict is not resolvable; there's no settlement to be had, but in confronting the unachievable object of desire there is what Lacan refers to as 'the game', following the logic of Freud's 'fort-da' (SE XVIII), of satisfying the pleasure principle as we engage with the non-specific objet a. So it is that we keep reading, reading for pleasure, the pleasure at least in part of being a serious, engaged reader of Literature (with a capital L). Each new text, each new author, each enlightened rereading, each new insight constitutes a move in the game. The game is never-ending, but that's where enjoyment lies.

In this serial process of identifications, we often engage with the subject in the form of a cathected figure, a person, an institution or product of some significant figure. The relations with this other are analogous to the relations with the analyst experienced by the analysand. Our special

English teacher, who seems to embody the ideal-ego we aspire to but who also, enigmatically, represents the subject's demanding otherness that impinges on our ego-ideal as an intense lack for as long as we fall short, as we must, as student-subjects, of the subject ideal.

Both recognition and misrecognition are intricated in this process. The subject is both 'free' and 'subjected' at the same time. I 'chose' English as 'my' subject, 'freely' subjecting myself. 'I' claim my free role in an autonomous decision-laden progress, enflamed by my 'natural' desire to be the incarnation of subject identity; but my passage into this position must be achieved through submission and obeisance to the Subject that stands as some mythical construct, some regulating, consistently organized other that can stand as an often enigmatic point of arbitration, if it comes to it, for my subjectivity within the Subject order. I am free to read Austen or Wordsworth or Beckett; I am free to follow F.R. Leavis, Northrop Frye, Jean Baudrillard or Terry Eagleton in my subject orientation; but I must demonstrate my inwardness with certain protocols for being an accredited bearer of subject identity. These include the address of literature, an understanding of language, an ability to write in standard form and to deploy a range of approved concepts for reading and interpretation. All of these vary in emphasis and in order of significance. The elements of the subject are held together by no clearly defined and articulable precepts or determined protocols. Rather, they held together by a modular logic that recognizes them as belong to the domain proper of the subject without having to either be consistent in their ethic, nor to speak to one another with any testable coherence. The Symbolic order of English is famously open and accommodating, a quality that makes it difficult to define, to grasp and to become inward with, being elusive and often depending on a nebulous 'feel' for things. In this the Lacanian perspective offers powerful insight, we believe, into the psychic processes at work in being interpellated through an educational order that is subtly pervasive and continuously demanding, ensuring both anxiety and jouissance as we engage with the call.

References

Others

Allen, A. (2016). Education, Mastery and the Marquis de Sade. *Other Education: The Journal of Educational Alternatives*, 5, 2.

Barthes, R. (1977). *Roland Barthes* (R. Howard, Trans.). Hill and Wang.

Bergey, B. W., & Ranellucci, J. (2025). How Early Pedagogical Experiences Relate to Teachers' Career Motivations. *Teaching and Teacher Education, 153*, 104808.

Beyond Ofsted. (2023). *An Inquiry into the Future of School Inspection Beyond Ofsted at a Glance.* https://beyondofsted.org.uk/wp-content/uploads/2023/11/Beyond-Ofsted-Executive-Summary.pdf

Bibby, T. (2011). *Education—An 'Impossible Profession'? Psychoanalytic Explorations of Learning and Classrooms.* Routledge.

Britzman, D. (1991). *Practice Makes Practice: A Critical Study of Learning to Teach.* SUNY Press.

Britzman, D. (2015). *A Psychoanalyst in the Classroom.* SUNY Press.

Clarke, M. (2019). *Lacan and Education Policy. The Other Side of Education.* Bloomsbury.

Clarke, M., & Kennedy, A. (2024). A Psychosocial Reading of Teacher Agency. *Teachers and Teaching*, 1–16. https://doi.org/10.1080/13540602.2024.2401090

Copjec, J. (2015). *Read My Desire. Lacan Against the Historicists.* Verso.

Creed, B. (1993). *The Monstrous-Feminine: Film, Feminism, Psychoanalysis.* Routledge.

DfE. (2019a). *Teacher Recruitment and Retention Strategy.* https://www.gov.uk/government/publications/teacher-recruitment-and-retention-strategy

DfE. (2019b). *Character Education Framework.* https://www.gov.uk/government/publications/character-education-framework

DfE (2021). *Teacher's Standards.* Guidance for school leaders, school staff and governing bodies. https://assets.publishing.service.gov.uk/media/61b73d6c8fa8f50384489c9a/Teachers_Standards_Dec_2021.pdf

DfE. (2022). *Political Impartiality in Schools.* https://www.gov.uk/government/publications/political-impartiality-in-schools/political-impartiality-in-schools

DfE. (2024). *Initial Teacher Training and Early Career Framework.* https://assets.publishing.service.gov.uk/media/65b8fa60e9e10a00130310b2/Initial_teacher_training_and_early_career_framework_30_Jan_2024.pdf

Dixon, J. (1967). *Growth through English.* National Association for the Teaching of English.

Eagleton, T. (1983). *Literary Theory: An Introduction.* University of Minnesota Press.

Ellis, V. (Ed.). (2024). *Teacher Education in Crisis: The State, the Market and the Universities in England.* Bloomsbury Academic.

Francis, B. (2008). Teaching Manfully? Exploring Gendered Subjectivities and Power via Analysis of Men Teachers' Gender Performance. *Gender and Education, 20*(2), 109–122.

Gorard, S., Maria Ventista, O., Morris, R., & See, B. H. (2023). Who Wants to be a Teacher? Findings from a Survey of Undergraduates in England.

Educational Studies, 49(6), 914–936. https://doi.org/10.1080/03055698.2021.1915751

Greteman, A. J. (2015). Corrupting Conversations with the Marquis de Sade: On Education, Gender, and Sexuality. *Studies in Philosophy and Education, 35*(6), 605–620.

Heinz, M. (2015). Why Choose Teaching? An International Review of Empirical Studies Exploring Student Teachers' Career Motivations and Levels of Commitment to Teaching. *Educational Research and Evaluation, 21*(3), 258–297.

Herbert, A. (2012). Pedagogy and the Gaze. In B. Bergstedt, A. Herbert, & A. Kraus (Eds.), *Initiating Learning* (pp. 19–34). Waxmann Verlag.

Hunter, I. (1994). *Rethinking the School: Subjectivity, Bureaucracy, Criticism* (1st ed.). Routledge.

Kristeva, J. (1982). *Powers of Horror: An Essay on Abjection.* Columbia University Press.

Lortie, D. (1975). *Schoolteacher: A Sociological Study.* University of Chicago Press.

Miller, J-A. (2009). Editorial. In *The Symptom*, 10.

Miller, J-A. (2013). From Symptom to Fantasy and Back. In *The Symptom*, 14.

Ofsted (2015). *Early Years Self-Evaluation Form* [Withdrawn]. https://www.gov.uk/government/publications/earlyyears-online-self-evaluation-form-sef-and-guidance-for-providers-delivering-the-early-years-foundation-stage

Ofsted. (2023). *Education Inspection Framework.* https://www.gov.uk/government/publications/education-inspection-framework

Ofsted. (2022). *Curriculum Research Review: English.* https://www.gov.uk/government/publications/curriculum-research-review-series-english/curriculum-research-review-series-english

Ormrod, J. (2014). *Fantasy and Social Movements.* Palgrave Macmillan.

Parker, I., & Pavón-Cuéllar, D. (2021). *Psychoanalysis and Revolution.* 1968 Press.

Peim, N. (2022). *Rethinking the Politics of Education.* Routledge.

Peim, N. (2024). *A Critique of Pure Education. Radically Rethinking the Education Archipelago.* Palgrave.

Priestley, M., Biesta, G., & Robinson, S. (2013). Teachers as Agents of Change: Teacher Agency and Emerging Models of Curriculum. *Reinventing the Curriculum: New Trends in Curriculum Policy and Practice, 20*, 187–206.

Priestley, M., Biesta, G. J. J., Philippou, S., & Robinson, S. (2015). The Teacher and the Curriculum: Exploring Teacher Agency. In *The SAGE Handbook of Curriculum, Pedagogy and Assessment* (pp. 187–201). University of Stirling.

Schutz, P. A., Crowder, K. C., & White, V. E. (2001). The Development of a Goal to Become a Teacher. *Journal of Educational Psychology, 93*(2), 299–230.

Stock, N. (2024a). Classroom Architecture and the Gaze. Beyond the Panopticon. *Discourse: Studies in the Cultural Politics of Education, 45*(4), 521–535.

Stock, N. (2024b). Fantasies of Rousseau: A Lacanian View of Natural Education in and Beyond Émile. *Educational Theory, 74*, 529–550.

Vick, M. J., & Martinez, C. (2011). Teachers and Teaching: Subjectivity, Performativity and the Body. *Educational Philosophy and Theory, 43*(2), 178–192.

Webster, J. (2022). *Disorganization and Sex.* Divided.

Žižek, S. (1998). Kant and Sade: The Ideal Couple. In *lacanian ink*, 13.

CHAPTER 4

On the Structures of Pedagogy

Abstract Teaching is reconsidered as a form of staging that is ordered by the idea of pedagogy as a powerful, though elusive, dimension of the Symbolic order of education. Is pedagogy as straightforward as the standard transmission and active engagement models suggest? Essentializing developmental models are put into question, and the easy assumption of the activation of pedagogy is approached through psychoanalytic rethinking of the dynamics of institutional space. The role of 'lack' is considered in terms of the teacher's experience of pleasure in teaching while the general order of knowledge is reviewed from a Lacanian perspective giving an emphasis to the interplay between discourse and incompletion. Finally, the role of the idea of potential is deliberated in relation to the dynamic function of lack in education while the governing role of education, through various 'points de capiton' gets foregrounded.

Keywords Pedagogy • Pedagogical relationship • Educational psychology • Learning • Teaching • Student • Potential • Progress • Memory understanding • Classroom • Theatre stage • Phallus • Lack • Knowledge • Paradigm • Point de capiton • Subject supposed to know

...psychoanalysis is ... first and foremost, a critique of pedagogy.
—Felman (1982, p. 23)

© The Author(s), under exclusive license to Springer Nature Switzerland AG 2025

N. Stock, N. Peim, *The Lacanian Teacher*, The Palgrave Lacan Series, https://doi.org/10.1007/978-3-031-93018-8_4

The Stage

When the teacher returns from the summer holiday, the first day, always a 'training' day, is full of the trading of terror in returning to the classroom. 'I've forgotten how to teach' we all say to one another. The forgetting in itself is interesting: for the simple acknowledgment that it has been forgotten implies that it has not really been forgotten, at least in any meaningful sense. As Freud makes clear in his vital essay ***Remembering, Repeating and Working Through*** (SE XII), remembering is only the first act of the psychoanalytic encounter, one that normally unconsciously hides what cannot be avowed. When the teacher 'forgets' how to teach, that is, remembering what it is like to be in the classroom, there is a peculiar disavowal of what teaching is. What is meant in their performative forgetting, we suggest, is that the teacher has forgotten how to be a teacher, how to pedagogise, how to occupy the space of that particular subject. A day or so after the training day, when classroom teaching is back in full swing, so comes the chorus of 'After a day back in the classroom it all came back to me!' We are reminded that the Symbolic space of the school, the locus of signifiers that we so thoroughly congregate around with teaching, allows the teacher to occupy that space once again with ease. This raises interesting questions, partly about pedagogy and partly about the Symbolic. What is forgotten? A set of techniques, procedure, rules? How to arrange the furniture? Or perhaps the nebulousness of pedagogy, it being a mode of deportment, means that, in absence, we risk losing touch with its requirements, its habits. That way of carrying oneself, the pedagogic modality of being, is itself a portion, perhaps, of the Symbolic order, with its own range of signifiers and its own grammar. Pedagogy, it seems, is less about knowing specific moves, than about managing intersubjective relations wherein roles are negotiated within a regime and fantasy is realised as a way of being in that world. Not so much a strict choreography, more a 'comportmental' *nous*.

One does not forget how to teach, but rather phases in and out of aspects of the Symbolic. In each phase, a staging of a certain form of desire takes place. We do not invoke the image of the stage here accidentally. Perhaps Lacan's most famous concept, 'the Mirror Stage' (discussed in Chap. 2), makes important wordplay with 'stage' that we wish to pause on at the start of this chapter. Of course, in Lacan's Freudian parlance, the stage he refers to is akin to that of a phase—a segment in the temporal that the subject passes through, much like the oral or phallic stages of psychosexual development (SE VII). Certainly, the educational implications are already clear here: that school is not only broken into phases or stages itself (in fact in England the years are broken into different 'Key Stages'), but that school is itself a stage or staging of one's life that one must pass through as a pivotal part of development as a subject, and that one must indeed 'act out'. Schools are obsessively concerned with other forms of staging: of learning, yes, but also of institutions with their differential Symbolic valency. From early years to primary; from higher to further; from state school to elite university; from school to the so-called real world, and so on. This positively oriented development of the stage of schooling and the logic of education we have spoken to much already in the previous three chapters, and in the close of this chapter we will look more closely at the punctuation that arrests this development—the 'point de capiton' as Lacan calls it (E, p. 303).

The Mirror Stage and the school stage, as temporal phases, are both implicated in the development of the ideal-ego, with resonances with other meanings to the signifier 'stage'. Lacan refers to not only a phase, but also a *stade*: the stage of a theatre, platform of performance, a stadium or arena. In this sense, the performance that takes place in the mirror of the Mirror Stage, the arena of one's subjectivation as an 'I' outlined in Chap. 2, is something that we can see occurring in the school. It is in the doubled 'stage' of schooling that both teachers and students alike must perform a certain ideal-ego on the stage of the great arena of educational competition. We are not being simply rhetorical here, and neither is Lacan. The *frame* of the mirror, either an actual frame or simply in its outline, gives the mirrored subject the appearance of a deliberately framed image, like a painting in a gallery or a picture on a screen.[1] So too does the subject perform in that mirrored image, just as subjects do within in the architecture of the theatrical stage or the arena. This is vital, as the social architecture of the classroom emulates the theatre:

> There is of course the actual screen at play of a projector or digital whiteboard, something that the students regularly watch and perhaps something that gazes at them. But the frame of the whiteboard also creates a screen like image. Even more so does the teacher, framed by the four corners of the

[1] In fact, Lacan makes a great deal of the frame in the dream of the Wolfman, Freud's famous case study where a man dreams he see wolves out of his window sitting in a tree. Lacan claims that 'the fantasy is framed' (X, p. 73); the desirable scene is only made so by its framing through the edging of the window.

> wall they teach from. Lecture halls often have a stage, once again with a backdrop of a massive screen or whiteboard. (Stock, 2024, p. 9)

If we take this to be the case, that the classroom is a theatrical space akin to the mirror or the screen, we might find further important resonances. The stage has rules that are bound to the script, though of course there is some room to manipulate the delivery of the script, and some characters even have license to go off script (once again we are reminded of the melancholic image of the Shakespearean fool in the primal scene of one author's teaching). This space is very similar to Lacan's subject and their mode of being in the Symbolic order. We receive lines from the big Other, then must enunciate them to play the part that we have little (conscious) control over. But the Real butts in, and we manipulate those lines, again often unbeknownst to ourselves, while Others on the stage might react in ways that the script could never have foreseen. There is even room for the psychotic break—in soliloquy to turn from the stage to the audience and expose it all as a sham. *But that's all one, our play is done, And we'll strive to please you every day* ... This, oddly perhaps, can be one of the ways of enhancing the 'authority' or 'veracity' of the teacher in the pedagogic scene, as one who can break with the role even while performing it confidently. One of us recalls a CSE folder lesson time one year, where a student chastised them for mucking about with another student, telling jokes or some such. 'Sir, come over here! This is proper fucking work!'

The classroom operates like any other stage, something highlighted by Roland Barthes in his essay on teaching with much reference to Lacan. Instances of actual scripting in lessons are becoming more common, with direct lines being given to (likely deskilled) teachers to ensure they cover the classroom content in a manner deemed acceptable to the politically motivated leadership of the school. The very notion of the lesson plan implies a script, if only a loose one with some moments of what we might think of as improvisation. But the teacher's script is inscribed in the Symbolic far more deeply than the ephemeral lesson plan. They are beholden to laws of speech that repeat the Symbolic order of educational impulses: Educate! No matter what, no matter how, is the script of the subject who inhabits the position of teacher in the classroom. As Barthes notes, 'the teacher escapes neither the theatre of speech nor the Law played out on its stage' (1977, p. 192). Thus to even enter the space of the classroom makes demands on the subject to become a teacher, to inhabit that Imaginary and Symbolic realm.

We cannot forget that the subject is always already in a relation to the Other, and in this staging, the audience, as students, are 'in the picture' (XI, p. 96) too. The audience in this case are not just an audience; they too are actors in the space, if not on the same stage. Like the stage of the radical playwright Bertolt Brecht, a figure we will return to, the actor plays a part that they have been placed within, not necessarily convincingly, and the audience in their distancing and estrangement [*Verfremdungseffekt*] are embroiled in the theatre as an extension to its space. The Brechtian audience is not a separate Other that can be enraptured by the actors on stage but rather another fragment of its illusory space. A closer attunement to this Brechtian space is essential for the reimagining of the teacher, as we aim to do in the final chapter, but his position of the theatrical nature of life chimes with Lacan's claims of the subject being represented by a signifier to another signifier (XI, p. 207)—a statement that positions everyone as costumed, scripted, and received by other actors.[2]

Extending beyond the teaching stage, the classroom is the space, or place, of education just as Lacan refers to at the beginning of *The Place, Origin and End of My Teaching*, 'the place I have come to, which puts me in a position to teach' (MT, pp. 4–5). As we have explored in the previous two chapters, the teacher who enters this space, both in terms of their structure as a subject and the fantasies that allow them to enter the place of teaching as teachers, here we turn our focus to the activities of classrooms that are bound to the space in which they occur. Though allusions have been made in the previous two chapters to some of the forms of enjoyment that exist for the teacher, this chapter will also look more

[2] This way of conceiving of the classroom has far-reaching philosophical antecedents, particularly when thinking of the space that engenders ways of being. Plato's concept of *Khôra* found in *Timaeus*, expanded by Derrida, is worth pausing on. What is *Khôra*? It's very difficult to define, to point to even and identify, but we know it's there. It's like the topology of the Lacanian Real, a space before space as we measure, read and experience it, the place of the place, the hollow of being that has to be populated, dressed up and animated—or it remains too frighteningly primordial. As Derrida says: 'Khora is not, above all not, a support or a subject which would give place by receiving or by conceiving, or even by letting itself be conceived. How can one deny it this essential signification of receptacle, when this very name is given to it by Plato? Difficult indeed. Perhaps we have not yet thought what it means to receive, the receiving of the receptacle' (Derrida, 1995, p. 95). Kristeva, following Derrida and drawing on Lacanian topology, goes a step further: 'Although the khôra can be designated and regulated, it can never be definitively posited: as a result, one can situate the khôra and, if necessary, lend it a topology, but one can never give it axiomatic form' (Kristeva, 1984, p. 26).

closely at the dominant forms of enjoyment that are engendered by the space of the classroom. If we describe this space, analogically, as the 'warped' space of education (warped in the same sense that any and every social space is warped in its own special way) that gives rise to the entities that inhabit it: its elements, its fundamental particles, forces, temporal movements and so on. In part, we raise the powerful effect the big Other's call has in the classroom in the forms of 'teaching and learning' compulsively enacted by teachers, particularly those that align themselves with the signifier of the curriculum. We also look at the relationships between teachers and students, shaped by certain Symbolic functions, that often have troublingly divisive effects invested in the enjoyment of the Other. Underscoring these classroom dimensions, we mainly focus here on the performance of the idealised classroom, the one that supposedly cuts through the neoliberal bureaucracy of contemporary education. This is the classroom that privileges pedagogy. Pedagogy is a conscious and unconscious concern of all teachers. It is, of course, in pedagogical terms that the most 'liberatory' forms of education are offered: as in the 'democratic' classroom or school (Watts, 1977). What we will work through in this chapter and the next, in correspondence with Lacan's graph of sexuation from Seminar XX, is how the pedagogical relationship does not exist, a fatal wound to the educational project of modernity that we outlined in Chap. 1.

Pedagogy in the Classroom

The Imaginary form of the classroom rests on the possibility of pedagogy to allow teaching to take place—and learning as its inherent but equally disturbing dialectical force. Indeed, it is in the Symbolic *relationship* posited by pedagogy that the script is written for the teacher. Pedagogy is a slippery signifier, often a substitution for education, teaching, learning, curriculum, and many other metonymically chained signifiers. It would be easy to attribute the idea of Lacanian 'master signifier' to pedagogy, a signifier that is without a referent that impels other chains of signification to take place (III, p. 268). This forecloses what the idea of pedagogy *does*, a signifier of the logic of relations in the classroom that upholds and structures its Symbolic space. Pedagogy also situates an *objet a* through its structural relationship—an inherently disappointing end to be reached in its terminus. There are certainly less positive associations with pedagogy as the disciplinary order of education, its framing. Where there is teaching there shall be a disciplinary relation, drawing on an order, an order that feeds back to the at once classificatory 'system of knowledge' (that we explore in due course) that is also at the same time and always a social relation (Bernstein, 1995). In general terms, however, a psychologistic discourse permeates the Symbolic relationship of pedagogy as we know it, foreclosing the disciplinary, social, classificatory function.

The modern project of education has exemplified a 'dependency on the field of psychology' (Britzman, 1991, p. 30), a consistent failure to position itself in its grafting onto another discourse. Pedagogy as we discuss it today is partially indebted to a narrow strain of educational psychology that not only rejects the unconscious in its origins, but has also been reduced and bowdlerized in its educational application. The classroom script we speak of is thus provided to us neatly by the likes of Piaget, Vygotsky, and increasingly Baddeley (discussed at later point in the chapter), as a linear path of student development. Piaget is regularly taught on teacher training courses, remains a firm favourite of educational psychologists, and generally forms the unconscious view of the student as a subject that teachers hold. This view maintains that the subject as a child is in a process of becoming that will 'unfold naturally if the student has enough empty space into which to grow' (Johnson, 2014, p. 3). They will grow, if the educational environment is appropriately staged, into a rational and autonomous agent—a fully formed subject. The classroom and accompanying educational spaces have been almost universally, albeit unconsciously, agreed upon as the space this can occur in. If the image the student sees on the Symbolic screen is the teacher (as become-complete), proffering the educational narrative that will fill the gap the student experiences, they will have learnt what there is to be learned. But Lacan's mirror stage and its inherent gaze troubles Piaget's narrative of progress in this sense by positing that the image of the teacher is only a fantasy. Lacan is unsurprisingly dismissive of Piaget's methods, highlighting.

> the futility of Piaget's child psychology. If you ask a child questions based on a logical apparatus [...] then it is scarcely surprising that you find this logical apparatus in the child you are questioning. You observe it there the moment it begins to bite, rises to the bait in the child, but to deduce from this that it is the child's development that constructs the logical categories ... (MT, p. 34)

Beyond his view of Piaget's methods is that the student, in the embrace of education, is seen as on a path to completion and wholeness, ascending a hierarchically staged path to reach a 'privileged area within the human field, defined as the field of people who have the singular ability to handle language' (p. 104), and in turn the teacher occupies this space of presence, solidity, and civility imagined for the child in the future. The subject is, if we remember, not present in the classroom as Piaget would have us believe. Rather, they always-partially present, cut by their unconscious and by their place as speaking-subject. The would-be Piagetian subject will always find themselves confronted with what Lacan calls castration, but we might simply restate as never finding themselves whole.

The pedagogical adoption of Piaget as classic learning theorist is echoed in the privilege accorded to Vygotsky as a champion of learning for social psychology. Invariably read as a linguistic functionalist, Vygotskyian thinking permeates educational discourses of learning. Teacher and learner are abstract positions engaged in a joint enterprise to address knowledge mediated by carefully manoeuvring through everyday thinking to the specialist terminology of scholastic knowledge that is equated with science. While this model, favoured by activity theorists and others, suspends any question of language in relation to social code, such as Bernstein (1975, 1995) might raise, it also forecloses the unconscious dimension, and never considers the 'incessant sliding of the signified under the signifier' in its wilful abstraction (E, p. 419). The Vygotskian subject, in its educational guise, invariably appears in a functionally positive dyad where the shared aim of learning is never interfered with by any contingent psychic material. What's more the more demotic 'zone of proximal development' [ZPD] (Vygotsky, 1978), a potentially radical idea, gets bowdlerized in educational discourses into a purely developmental space for learning's accumulative progress (Edwards and Daniels, 2004). ZPD's potency as mode of '"unthought", a more radical ontological meaning' (Peim, 2009, p. 177) has traces of Lacan's Real or unconscious, but of course these possibilities are foreclosed in the enfolding of it back into the Symbolic relationship of pedagogy. The ZPD is a space only to be filled with knowledge 'delivered' through pedagogy.

This psychologically inflected discourse manifests more mundanely as classroom pedagogy. It is the premise, so it goes, that teachers must be able to attend to gaps in students' knowledge so to allow them to progress, something we will explore in more detail in the conclusion of this chapter. This is not to say that the teacher is the one who has to fill the gap (and this is where 'critical' forms of pedagogy intervene to be examined in the next chapter), nor that knowledge has to be purely instrumental. In simplest terms, pedagogy is this teacher/student relation, and it is the dimension that makes teaching enjoyable for many educators. Beyond this, it is a condition for the teaching/learning relationship that says the teacher is to attend to the gap in the being of the student, a gap that is not just an absence or lack of knowledge, but a socio-ontological gap (pardon the expression) that demands all the 'framing' pedagogical activity that attends specific teaching. This is the inherited model of education as essential social apparatus that expresses an essential social good. This now embedded, received idea comes from, in part at least, the ethic of childhood that now prevails, and that gets extended into the 'pedagogized society' (Bernstein, 1995). Emil Cioran, from a purely pessimistic point of view, makes a similar claim in dehistoricized form that 'Since Adam men's entire effort has been to modify *man*' through the 'aims of reform and pedagogy' (2018, p. 26). This apparently ancient logic, that Foucault demonstrated as the key to understanding biopower in modernity (Foucault, 1991), extends far beyond the classroom, though the irony that Cioran identifies foreshadows what we will go on to discuss: man 'subsists unchanged' (p. 27), but as Foucault might put it, can be trained to appear in the guise of a pre-designed template. Lacan is peculiarly relevant here because of the ontological dimension of his thinking around the 'hole', the 'want-to-be' and the ontological importance of recognition in the field of social identity (Miller, 2006) that we tackle here and previously.

A typical classroom encounter for the English teacher might be framed through this pedagogical relationship—teaching Shakespeare to a class of teenagers—with the intended purpose of being able to analyse the use of extended metaphors in the language so to develop understanding of both character and style. The class are given an extract from the play they have been studying, *The Tempest,* and an interchange between Sebastian and Antonio, two typically corrupt royals pursuing power. Sections like these can cause great pains to some students. They may find the language impenetrable, the point of the scene abstruse, may have forgotten who the minor characters involved are, may not be familiar with the stylistic features, and inevitably respond with 'I don't get it'. 'Which bit don't you get?' the dutiful pedagogue replies, zeroing in on the misunderstanding to correct it, their enjoyment starting to bubble in the situation of knowing what the student asks to know. 'All of it, I don't get any of it.' The enjoyment starts to fade, seeing the student unable to even identify what they misunderstand. What a failure the pedagogue has been up to this point, unable to even make the simplest of extended metaphors reveal themselves to the student. No matter, the enjoyment can be refound. More questions follow: 'Do you understand what Sebastian means in the first line?' 'Do you remember what Antonio's relationship to the King is?' 'What do you think Sebastian wants of Antonio?' 'What does it mean when the key word is this or that?' And so on and so on. The enjoyment froths as the student starts to claim they understand, 'Now I get it, yeah, I get it.' The student now understanding the metaphor, the pedagogue's duty has been fulfilled. But it is in a simple exchange like this we find the seeds of pedagogical impossibility and its intertwining with, what we will say is, following Lacan, a jouissance of belief in a signifier of non-lack. As Lacan demands 'Where is understanding when we understand, when we think we understand?' (VIII, p. 197). Exchanges like these, micro-pedagogical encounters so common to the teacher, are replete with the question of where the understanding of the object being studied lies. Lacan's answer is revealing and deals a fatal wound to pedagogy.

> I posit that, in its surest and, I daresay elementary form, our understanding of anything the subject tells us can be defined at the conscious level, by the fact that we know how to respond to what he demands. It is insofar as we think we can respond to his demand that we have the sense that we understand. (VIII, p. 197)

This is the starting point for all those liberalised practices of English teaching (Dixon, 1967; Barnes, 1976; Britton, 1970) and teaching in general (Holt, 1990) that seek to displace the direct teacher/student encounter through the practices of group work that 'enable' the students to articulate, in their 'own' idiom, their response and inchoate understanding in the required subject idiom. The demand the pedagogue consciously hears from the student to explain the metaphor is not the demand unconsciously made by the student—to be allowed to forget Sebastian and Antonio forever more, say. 'Demand is not explicit' (VIII, p. 197), but it must be for the functionality of the pedagogue and for the pedagogue's enjoyment. This is not just in the quotidian classroom, but recurs in various forms. In Activity theory, for instance, the bold claim is made that any social activity can be rendered as a pedagogic space. The role of the 'activity theorist' is to provide the pedagogic occasion so that all involved in the activity, a whatever level, might contribute to its reinscription as a more functional unit, firmly focussed on its collective goal (Engeström, 2003). A trip to the cinema or a chat in the pub is here enfolded into pedagogy; the big assumption of this social pedagogy is that the collective goal—of improving the 'service'—is collectively shared and isomorphic. There is no possible allowance for desire, for the unconscious, for jouissance. These untidy and unconscious dimensions would ruin the pedagogic fantasy of rationally achieved, collectively agreed improvement.

Nevertheless, the way the pedagogue thinks he understands allows for the possibility of attenuating misunderstanding. In an inverse fashion, this (mis)understanding of what the student demands actually places a demand on the student, 'to give something that satisfies the expectation of the educator' (VIII, p. 203). In this quotation from Seminar VIII, Lacan talks of the demand the parent places on the child to hold in their excrement so to satisfy the parent in their call for toilet training. This anality is perhaps not so different from what we see in pedagogy, as it allows for the enjoyment to occur when the child 'holds it in' and then 'evacuate[s]' (p. 203) for their own pleasure. Such anality certainly pervades many layers of education, including the demand for students to retain vast amounts of 'knowledge' to be evacuated on the page in an exam. Some teachers even use phrases like 'knowledge dump' to indicate how an exam should be started. While such an evacuation may be a quite minor form of pleasure for the student, it is certainly a highly deferred pleasure for the teacher. But the form of enjoyment, or to use Lacan's term 'jouissance' (discussed in more detail in Chaps. 5 and 6) at play in pedagogy, is an enjoyment that stretches beyond and is different from 'mere' pleasure, particularly in the Shakespeare example above. Jouissance is a mode of pleasure that includes some uncertainty, anxiety even, and experiences the object of desire, say full knowledge and understanding of the text in our example above, as deferred, as perhaps glimpsed at through some intermediary object of phenomenon, a partial insight, a transliteration into contemporary vernacular, say. In this sense it is 'what serves no purpose' (XX, p. 3), as it extends beyond the neat arrangement of satisfaction from having taught something or the pleasurable feeling of being liked by your students (or so you believe). Jouissance is fraught with a tension that touches on some quite far-reaching dimensions of one's being. While proffering the possibility of mastery, jouissance is to be had in its non-realizable anticipation. This is something we will explore further in the final chapter.

The Signifier of Lack

So what is the mode of enjoyment, or jouissance, for the pedagogue? What we care to venture is that jouissance so regularly experienced by the teacher in any pedagogical practice—any classroom practice—is what Lacan refers to as 'phallic jouissance' (XX, p. 7), or enjoying attenuating lack. We use the term phallus carefully and need to lay some groundwork to explore it properly, as some might rightly recoil at the notion of 'the phallus' being central to the project of education or perceive it to be an androcentric term. Lacan is aware of this, but it is precisely its androcentrism that Lacan diagnoses as a structural condition of the subject in the Symbolic order. We also choose to use the term 'signifier of lack' predominantly, as it is exactly this that Lacan is getting at. Let us explain further.

We may know of the ostensibly sexist theory of Freud's regarding penis envy (SE XIX), that little boys one day discover they have a penis which becomes a great source of anxiety for them in the fear of castration by their parents, whereas little girls encounter the penis and envy it due to their lack. This process is tied to the Oedipus complex, to castration anxiety, and to the often-phallic readings of dreams we might think of in stereotypes of psychoanalysis (though these stereotypes are often very far from Freudian dream analysis and there is much more to Freud than just Oedipus). But Lacan once again offers an interesting reformulation of Freudian thought. Rather than penis envy, referencing the biological appendage, Lacan switches emphasis to the phallus, that is to what exists within the Imaginary and the Symbolic (not the penis) as a *signifier* (E, p. 579) and a signifier of lack. The Imaginary and Symbolic manifestation of the phallus is vital, reminding that the appearance of it (in its various forms) in sexuality, discourse, and relationships, are a product of language, a clear example being the use of the phallus as the signifier of sexual difference (E, p. 576). There is no Real phallus or power to it either, although the patriarchal structures of the Symbolic world might have us believe that there is.

As such the phallus is the signifier imbued with power that inherently signifies a lack in the Other—*our lack*. This is not just in its absurd positioning as the erect image of domination that we might think of in caricatures of Freudian dream analysis (a tower, a train going into a tunnel, a piston, and so on), but rather substantiated by its veiling (E, p. 512). The recoil that we might feel in even mentioning the phallus is a further inscription of its power. So too with knowledge, which seems out of reach, hidden by the veil of the academy, the library, the archive, the teacher ... And yet, despite its correlate to power, it is a signifier that only exists in the Symbolic relation to other, lacking signifiers. We cannot *be* or *have* signifiers; we may adorn ourselves with them as some masque of lack, but they are not possessed by us (instead belonging to the big Other). The signifier of lack is not and cannot be held by anyone; it is impotently grasped at in the formations of desire, but in its position as a master signifier, it remains elusive and unobtainable.

Everyone is wounded by this lack, no matter how much that some people might believe they are not. Indeed, any time one believes that they 'complete' another, they are in belief of possessing the signifier of lack (E, p. 472). We might remember that a lack, or cut, is essential to theory of the Lacanian subject. Lacan is thus not invested in revealing or substantiating the phallus, but rather seeks to decentre, or perhaps even deconstruct it, at least to reveal its mythical ontological status. What he does identify in the subject, however, is how the phallus as shorthand for a signifier of lack has a structural hold on being: the Symbol of that which when obtained might complete lack, it becomes a master signifier of any desirable object. The links between lack and knowledge are becoming clearer, and as such are coupled with the formation of pedagogy. Lacan's claim that 'it is more precious to hold onto desire's symbol ... than to hold onto desire itself' (VIII, p. 229) is telling. We would rather pursue the completion to be obtained by some dimension of non-lack, which could be say knowledge, consciousness, Enlightenment, redemption, and so on, than to pursue our own desires. To enter into the structural relationship of pedagogy is thus, on some level, to offer non-lack to another through the desire for knowledge.

The order of knowledge is always a signifier of lack in the Other—we who are seeking it, always, however obliquely or arcanely, making reference to some putative but unreachable, undefinable object that holds the order of things in place and that determines the hierarchic structure of being education represents, enacts and reproduces. Lacan makes the bold claim that 'it is no longer possible to play the role suitable for the transmission of knowledge without being a psychoanalyst' (XVI, p. 137). There are many ways of interpreting this intentionally provocative statement. We might read it as Lacan tracing both the psychoanalyst's awareness of the impossibility of transmission, or perhaps the reframing of teaching as an impotent grasp for non-lack. Both pose the question of the order of knowledge, that in some far-reaching way, determines the pedagogic relation, both in its various Imaginary and idealized modes and in its mundane practice. This order of knowledge is manifest in all sorts of perhaps unlikely places as well as in the obvious ones, such as the university faculty office. Through university and school curricula, now universalized, it gets distributed, albeit in diffuse form. This non-lacking dimension of knowledge makes sense of the fact that the apparently arbitrary attainment of position in the hierarchical order can carry an authority way beyond the personal attributes of the holder of the position.

Knowledge thought of in this way, as 'expert' and held by a privileged few afforded to them by the institutions of education, is in part what Lacan refers to as the discourse of the university (XVII, p. 148). Often the university discourse is discussed in its political stewarding of the master's discourse (Clarke, 2019, p. 74)—that is, as upholding the quasi-feudal position of authoritarian rule over subjects.[3] University discourses of knowledge seek 'to soothe and sedate disquiet with the reassuring confidence of objective knowledge' (p. 73), something that will continue to become clear in this chapter in our considerations of knowledge. However, there is more to examine in terms of the way knowledge operates *as* educational, for the purposes of pedagogy, alongside its stewardship of the master. Consider, for instance, a university department of English where the head of department is an expert on Shelley, has edited recent collections of Shelley's work, including detailed textual commentary, and has done extensive exploratory work on the sources of Shelleyan ideas, phrases and cadences. This head of department is highly specialized, is primarily a scholar and not so much a critic (in the parlance of academic English), has scant knowledge of Piers Plowman, of the novels of James Joyce or the eighteenth-century essay. These elements of subject identity, along with myriad others, may be addressed (or not) by colleagues in the department who occupy less elevated positions. The point is not so much about

[3] The master's discourse takes the form of the 'pedicle' (XX, p. 31), a stem or a stalk, one that poses a possibility of something's being, an 'if'. It is 'quite simply being at 'someone's' heel, being at someone's beck and call – what would have been if you had understood what I ordered you to do' (p. 31). In this logic, education is the way that it is because it is what we (teachers, learners, managers, and so forth) have understood if we were ordered to do so. Nobody has given any such order; simply this is what we would have done were we ordered. 'Every dimension of being is produced in the wake of the master's discourse … the signifier commands' (p. 32). The master's signifier thus impels education to be as it is, and what is this master's signifier but 'education' itself. Educate! Educate now! We find this same point is made in relation to the big Other *as* education and its phallic signifier.

English as a subject that is, in Bernstein's (1975) terms, a 'collection code' but more to indicate that the authority of the head of department, who may be called upon to make crucial decisions defining the orientation of the department's research and scholarship, who will be expected to have a decisive hand in the appointment of colleagues, in their disciplining where 'necessary', and who will in general be expected to account for the standing of the department, to manage its everyday operations, its allocation of resources, its distribution of subject material across the now-common modular structure, who will be required to answer for the success of the department in degree examination results, in recruitment of higher level students and the rate and quality of production of published research, all a signifier of lack.

English, as an academic subject, then, has no centre, no determinate and co-ordinating principle, text or position. It exists, in the university, within a structure that identifies both it and its archons as being possessed with an authority derived from its being, in a non-lacking sense, both consistent and authoritative. Lacan is quite aware of this, of course, particularly in his regular allusion to knowledge reduced to the form of 'course credits' (XVI, p. 138) and university discourse (XVII)—arguably signifiers of an (Imaginary) obtainable, graspable thing. English degree courses vary enormously in universities across the world and even in those contexts that carry the most prestigious instantiations of it. Of course, there will be similarities and cross-overs and many points in common. As degree courses became more modularized, however, the central essence of subjects (such as English)—always open to some form of difference, dispute and contest—can be held in abeyance. The coherence of any English degree course and its consistency with Imaginary identification are legitimately held in play without being tied to any specific anchoring point. The structural temporality of this condition is perhaps worth commenting on as one cannot point to any point of origin as the defining and centring anchor. A qualified and established archon of the subject, our head of department, for instance, may insinuate some new element of subject practice into his repertoire of teaching or knowledge, as happened frequently in the 1970s and 1980s with ideas from what then described as post-structuralism, ideas that might shift practices, introduce new texts, open onto new objects of enquiry such as media texts and other elements of popular culture. Should such practices, that now carry the authority imbued by our non-lacking archon, take hold, others may come along and derive their own authority from these practices and forms of knowledge that had hitherto never been deemed as belonging to subject identity.

Much like the 'ancient mysteries' (E, p. 581) imbued in the signifier of the lack, a certain aura of the sacred may yet attach to certain elements of Imaginary identitification. They will be seen to be beyond the play of differences activated by the movement between what's established and what's deemed to be legitimately innovative. The aura of the knowledge of the university, that is, the knowledge pursued in the process of education, makes promises of emancipating the subject (only of course to do quite the opposite) (McGowan, 2013, p. 72). But even sacred objects may be subject to reformation and even to deformation, as has been the case with Shakespeare. Again, in the 1980s a series of influential texts written by established academics in the field of English addressed Shakespeare anew. No longer seen as the repository of eternal truths and essential insights in the human condition 'political Shakespeares' appeared (Dollimore & Sinfield, 1985; Drakakis, 1985). The sacred aura of the Shakespearean text was displaced by a critical analysis of ideas embodied in those texts that were seen as ripe for critique. The texts could be revisited as historical documents revealing, in the histories of their representation, the dominant ethic of the time that produced them. The very phenomenon of Shakespeare could be reinterpreted from a cultural, historical perspective to reveal new truths about the social significance of both cultural and educational practices. In addition, Shakespeare could be wilfully read as modern, as already bearing the truth of post-structuralist insight with uncanny prescience or with the application of techniques of reading that redefined the essential text. A 'new' cadre of archons could arise attaining academic reputations from engaging with these perspectives that would have been unthinkable in earlier incarnations of English. Roland Barthes once commented, in relation to the question 'What is Literature?' that troubled literary studies for a while, that 'Literature is what gets taught' (quoted in Eagleton, 1983, p. 194). The subject, then, and the (often very significant) social authority it claims is not founded in a specific substance or attributes.[4]

The point here, however, is to account for the process whereby knowledge that supports an institutional structure bearing far-reaching social

[4]Any Wittgensteinian might retort that this merely demonstrates the insight of their cynosure that practices belong together by 'family resemblances' rather than properties in common; so, of course we should not expect academic subjects to display coherence and consistency. But it is in the representation and in the management of fields of knowledge that insights into the phallic dimension of knowledge structures may be revealed beyond the ken of any Wittgensteinian.

effects, including, crucially, the distribution of identities in the social division of labour, is held to be authoritative and consistent, even though perhaps obscurely so. It is for this reason, amongst others, that Lacan calls for any teacher to be a psychoanalyst, that is, someone who 'takes seriously the question of the dependence of the subject on the discourse that has a hold on him and not that he proffers' (XVI, p. 138).

Without the function of a signifier of lack, English could not stand as such an authoritative body of 'knowledge' holding an absolutely central authority on the curriculum licenced to make daily judgments about the competence of native speakers, about the 'quality' and level of their speech and cultural competence. The principle of recontextualization means that the ubiquitous school curriculum—the legally ensconced national curriculum—that sets in at an ever earlier phase of life, draws on the very structure of authority that pertains at the level of the now global university (Bernstein, 1975). Every English teacher draws their classroom authority as a purveyor of subject identity from this nebulous but powerfully invested system. Everyone within the field of English—teachers, pupils, students, researchers, Shelley scholars—stands in some relation of deficit to this shifting but endowed order. This is the non-lacking dimension. The professor of English at the Russell group university who is a renowned specialist in Shelley may be considered well-endowed in relation to others: students, for instance, or lower order colleagues, and via the mythical figure of Shelley may be considered as the holder of a specific kind of lack filling truth, but even s/he must accede to the greater Symbolic order of things. This structure of course pertains to any and all disciplines, in any subject of the subject.

This starts to bring us back to the relationship implicit in pedagogy in terms of who holds the signifier of lack, that which is 'coveted by the subject' (E, p. 589). The English school teacher is deemed by pupils, and perhaps by their parents and colleagues, to be endowed with knowledge about the examination system, about the requirements of the syllabuses and how to teach and apply to the criteria of assessment—covetable objects in the Symbolic order of education. Indeed, within the context of the school, endowment affords the teacher a certain power rooted in subject knowledge and pedagogic know-how. But the teacher, transposed to another context of English, the University, say, will feel the lack of the kind of puissance enjoyed by the established figures within subject Symbolic order. This feature of knowledge contextualization is interesting in education, especially in relation to what Bernstein has referred to as 'recontextualization' and has an important bearing on our Lacanian account of the structure of authority and knowledge within and across institutions (Bernstein, 1975). The classroom teacher, teaching a limited range of texts, without the need to produce groundbreaking research or to make a decisive contribution to scholarship, both draws on subject authority and lacks it at the same time, having made a settlement with the symbolic order that grants some modicum of non-lacking status and that also may provide material support.

The subject English (or any other), then, is not an ontologically consistent entity. It is a master signifier instigating a metaphorical and metonymic chain across contexts of difference but retains a relation to an order that is also imbued with authority and grants identities in relation to its explicit and implicit judgments. All of this is held together by an authority that engages with the differentiated desire of its subjects—something that Lacan is again alluding to in his outline of the university discourse (XVII). No doubt the professor of English at the Russell group university will experience desire in relation to international reputation within the field. The new year eleven student in a British secondary school may desire a good result in her recent *Macbeth* test, while the reception infant just beginning school may not yet experience desire in relation to curriculum English, but will be encouraged to activate desire to become a 'free-reader' and to be granted a 'pen-licence'. Even the auto-didact, supposedly free from the constraints of the educational apparatus, may subject themselves to the pursuit of non-lacking authority found in the knowledge to be obtained in the pile of books on their table. Subject authority and pedagogy align in this constant process of engendering desire and positioning subjects with decisive judgements falling not only on performance but also on levels of desire and effective submission to the authority of the subject. Whether that orients around Shelley or the pen-licence, it does not matter.

From Signifier of Lack to Knowledge

Lacan's conceptualisation of the signifier of lack and its relation to knowledge has far reaching implications for epistemology, the philosophical canon, and of course pedagogy. In a significant extension of the epistemological stance, that, since Plato, problematizes certainty in knowledge[5] in order to establish grounds for it, the problematization of knowledge itself

[5] See for example *Meno*, Descartes, Hume … even Nietzsche.

is central to the psychoanalytic project (Grene, 1966; Moran, 2000; Peim, 2018). If we return to the Freud paper raised in the opening of the book, 'Wild Psychoanalysis' (SE XI), the biggest takeaway for those outside of the clinic is that knowledge cannot liberate the mind. If anything, the pursuit of knowledge only serves to shore up resistances and confirm preconceptions. Generally, the 'Promethean discovery' (E, p. 201) of psychoanalysis—the unconscious—necessitates the idea that we cannot even know ourselves, so how do we hope to gain knowledge of the Other? Felman, drawing on Lacan's Seminar II and XX in particular, makes this point in much greater detail:

> ...the unconscious, in Lacan's conception, is precisely the discovery that human discourse can by definition never be entirely in agreement with itself, entirely identical to its knowledge of itself, since, as the vehicle of unconscious knowledge, it is constitutively the material locus of a signifying difference from itself.
>
> What, indeed, is the unconscious, if not a kind of *unmeant knowledge* which escapes intentionality and meaning, a knowledge which is spoken by the language of the subject (spoken, for instance, by his 'slips' or by his dreams), but which the subject cannot recognize, assume as *his*, appropriate; a speaking knowledge which is nonetheless denied to the speaker's knowledge? (1982, p. 28)

There is no such thing as absolute knowledge, and this is not just a claim of the psychoanalysts. Just as Derrida indicated that science could not be immune from spectrality (1994) (the movement of the trace as disturbance to pure presence), so too Lacan, while acknowledging that science is a distinct mode of knowledge with a specific form of relation to 'Nature', interferes in his thinking, both explicitly and implicitly, with any association of science with necessary progress, teleology or historical necessity and certainly eschews any notion that science and scientific thinking means redemption from superstition (E, p. 726). This stands in contrast to a dominant strand in western thinking that is often found on the shelves of popular science books. Perhaps it is most obviously and popularly expressed in Bill Bryson's *History of Nearly Everything*. The 'nearly' in the title indicates the irritating gap indicating Bryson's longing to plug the various lacunae in scientific knowledge that prevent science from achieving a mastery of everything. The book offers a celebration of science's achievements but is at the same time harried by anxieties about its breakdowns, absences, incompletions. Bryson's anxieties, unable to cope with these aporia without the promise of future resolution, cheerfully anticipate resolution when the gaps will be filled and the modern subject of science complete, misreading, in effect, the role of those very gaps in knowledge that turn out to be the very conditions for the being of science. We are also reminded once again of the teacher outlined in Chap. 2 that must possess a subject, that is, demonstrate a total mastery of that subject for the demand of the students.

In relation to Lacan's thinking the question concerning science returns us to awkward questions concerning the truth not only of specific scientific discourses, but also of the role that science (as paradigm model of knowledge) plays in the order of the world of modern knowledge, especially in its curriculized form, the form that increasingly occupies education at all levels. As such, the following section, whilst complicated, is vital in thinking through the domain of knowledge in the educational Symbolic.

Lacan demonstrates a psychoanalytically informed rethinking of science in science's particular relation to beings, and its will to distinguish itself from metaphysics. Lacan introduces the third dimension of the subject that resonates with Bruno Latour's remodelling of the scientific order in his insistence that it is at the level of the subject that science is to be most properly understood (Latour, 1988). Lacan, like Latour, dispenses with the residue of logical positivism's[6] triumphant vision of a new relation to the truth of things and to thinking—whereby the subjective dimension was offset by objective modes of verification to clinch the security stability of scientific knowledge. As he says, 'logical positivism [is] in search of the "meaning of meaning"' (E, p. 416), with its insistence on objectivity via repeatability and testing, science fulfilled at one level the fantasy of a pure rationality, one grounded in the really Real, empirically verified and computable, overseen by the sovereign authority of (subjectless) mathematics. Indeed, 'Only mathematical algorithms resist this process; they are considered to be devoid of meaning, as they should be' (p. 416). Equations, it was discovered could (like magic formulae) unravel the truths, the secrets, indeed, of nature that had hitherto been shrouded in myth.

But it couldn't end there. While science could and did make reference to observable facts repeatedly tested for verification, the purely rationalist

[6]A philosophy that claims to dispense with metaphysics, logical positivism believes that philosophical problems that cannot be solved through the process of formal logic are not 'real' problems. It purports to be purely empirical and thus disavows the role of the subject, something that Lacan and others reinsert.

view foreclosed the historical dimension that acknowledged the equally compelling facts of scientific revolutions. Large scale changes in the understanding of things, often quite fundamental things: Darwin/Wallace in biology, Copernican and Einsteinian revolutions in astronomy, revealed science as subject to volcanic upheavals. There is no 'normal' condition for science, no metaphysics-free procedurality, only in a provisional sense that Thomas Kuhn (1970) came to refer to famously as a 'paradigm'.[7] The paradigm has a certain ambiguity: it holds existing knowledge together, while demanding, albeit within its own parameters, the production of new knowledge. Disruption of the paradigm, revolutionary, or more local, threatens conflict, even schism, and this especially becomes apparent in those domains of science that rely heavily on speculation verified by mathematical calculation. The norms that enfold the paradigm cannot be taken for eternal truths—to do so would be unscientific. Anomalies trouble the idea of a completed field of knowledge. Through generational change contested knowledge may become established, paradigms may be modified displaced or overthrown. There is no supreme court to determine cases in dispute and as Kuhn, whose ideas we roughly summarize here, affirms, there are forces of commitment and faith at stake in all of this. Just like Lacan's model, the subjectivity of the subject cannot be erased (Kuhn, 1970).

Kuhn's modelling makes explicit reference to the social dimension of both modest changes and paradigm shifts in science, or as Miller refers to it in the notes for *Écrits*, an 'epistemological break' (E, p. 852). What gets accepted as orthodoxy is likely to be influenced by key, established figures in the field accepting new knowledge or new models. Major changes in science are not, Kuhn implies, driven by purely scientific factors, deflating the image of science as uncontaminatedly disinterested or as a desire free-zone, impervious to the machinations of the unconscious. There is an 'epistemological drive' (E, p. 737) at play, and what's more, the direction and mode of scientific change indicate no necessarily linear progression. Even 'data' is determined to be theory-laden and inflected with desire.

[7] A set of fundamental theoretical assumptions/'laws', a set of exemplary problems or issues crying out for resolution, agreed methods for determining the dividing line between fact and speculation (never very clearly settled): while these things may prevail, they do so historically and change. And, of course, the other side of historicity is future orientation. Scientific discovery and revelation must include the unpredictable and must be predicated on the endless demand for the production of new knowledge designed to modify, refine, in some cases revolutionize existing, confirmed, scientific knowledge.

Data, delved from the Real, bears meaning relative to the paradigm: a basic unit of truth is always already determined by the symbolic order's organization of its engagement with the Real.

Kuhn refers to different scientists living in different worlds, echoing Lacan's famous toilet doors imagery (E, p. 416): where you are is not a function merely of geography. Although not acknowledged, Kuhn's thinking strongly influenced Foucault's account of the 'episteme' as a form of ruling order of knowledge (Foucault, 1977). The big shifts in knowledge, in Foucault's implicit view, cannot be understood independently of shifts in the social order. Science can't be abstracted from its apparatuses: including its ordering of identities, its embedded practices and, massively, its discourse that 'creates the objects of which it speaks'. Science, is, whatever else it is, of the order of the signifier.

And yet the idea of certain knowledge haunts thinking today, in centres dedicated to knowledge pursuit and production, as well as in what we might call a more generalized Symbolic order. There is an important paradox here in terms of what Freud declared blows to the 'self-love' of 'man' (sic) (SE XIV, p. 74). While science bristles with the confidence of demonstrative authoritative knowledge existing independently of hieratic charisma, at the same time, scientific knowledge displaces the centrality of the human: the Darwinian version of evolution introduces both a blind impersonal process in the emergence of species; the cosmological perspective decentres the earth as centre of creation and offers the nullifying promise of solar death as the ultimate telos.

While the emergence of modern science and enlightenment may have initially held out the promise of endless material earthly progress, negative possibilities necessarily attend to the drastically changed world order they inaugurated. The title page of Bacon's *Novum Organum* (1902) represents a ship of hope navigating the Pillars of Hercules into uncharted waters beyond. The opening onto new worlds, the great age of 'discovery', however, also signals the violent occupation, domination and exploitation (not yet exhausted) of lands and peoples by European powers. Science, enlightenment and the triumphs of rationality are accompanied by and accompany brutal conquest and destruction (Hochschild, 1998). Positive ideas about progress later had to confront and the Promethean discovery of the unconscious. Freud gloomily pondered the implacable death drive (SE XVIII), although unable to accommodate himself to its full implications. Copernicus had decentred the earth's position in creation. Einstein's revision of Newton made the world and its environs a much less stable place, and twentieth century cosmology, often regarded as the ultimate science, produced images of an increasingly vast and incomprehensible universe driven by contradictory forces that made uncertainty a defining principle and that increasingly acknowledged its own dependence on speculation to secure its narratives.[8] Though the classroom teacher may not believe themselves to be the master of knowledge, the student often perceives them as such to engender the relation. The teacher may still believe the student can come to master knowledge through the power of pedagogy.

What does all this have to do with classroom pedagogy, then? Even the humblest classroom practitioner, plying their pedagogic trade in the everyday classroom, partakes of the order of knowledge alluded to sketchily above. The great educational archipelago is threaded together into vast portion of the Symbolic order of knowledge, research and learning. The Symbolic order of education decrees what counts as knowledge and who counts as a purveyor of knowledge bearing whatever social symbolic value and institutional status that accrues to them through the Symbolic order. What's more that Symbolic order codes, practices, comportments and habits of thought of subjects within. As we hope to have illustrated in the previous chapter, the desire of the teacher—whatever form it may take—is generated in relation to the Symbolic and Imaginary order of education. The daily life of the teacher is replete with the signifiers of this order in the most mundane terminology of educational practices: assessment, grades,

[8] There is also powerful resonance to be found in the late contemporary of Lacan's, Jean Francois Lyotard. He privileged narrative as necessarily indicating the cultural dimension in knowledge forms including science, opening again question concerning genres of knowledge and the grounding of their authority (Lyotard, 1979). For Lyotard, narrative is associated with the overriding ideas or principles that govern modes of knowledge—most often unconsciously. The phrase 'grand narrative' signals a dominant world view or 'ethic'. Forms of knowledge have their roots in specific anthropological contexts, 'forms of life' organized in 'petits-recits' or small-scale language games. Lyotard's case challenges all positions that claim a privileged relation to reality—as though there could be forms of knowledge (science would be the paradigm case for our world) that could be uncontaminated by the socio-anthropological dimension. Lyotard points out that while science may claim to be free of such contamination, in fact, it must be organized as a system by narrative knowledge as much as by cool ratiocination or by neutrally construed 'method'. Nevertheless, science as neutral persists as a key idea in research including social science research. It is clear that in this assumption of a special relation to the real claimed for science with its suppression of narrative there must be a powerful element of fantasy that grants to science a certain powerfully mythologized phallic power.

curriculum, syllabus, lesson, subject, classroom, level … all draw from the world order of education as an authoritative and authorizing source of being and action. It is perhaps here we might understand what Lacan means in his enigmatic statement that 'Knowledge is something that was invented by pedagogues' (XVI, p. 173). Knowledge *must* be imagined in a certain way so to allow the teacher to believe themselves to be able to correctly disseminate it.

Recent policy reforms around teacher training emphasise the idea of a pure model of knowledge with regular references in such policy to the policy being 'based on the best available evidence' (DfE, 2024, p. 4) and drawing on 'feedback from a broad range of experts from across the education sector' (p. 4) (or, perhaps, state-nominated experts say Ellis & Childs, 2024, p. 5). Coupled with its formal element of pages of references to 'research', 'Much of the research included in the reference list is underpinned with scientistic assumptions about educational inquiry, and what constitutes the best available educational knowledge' (Hordern & Brooks, 2023, p. 811). Both the formal documentation *and* the counterarguments against from the academy are positioned in relation to 'research', 'knowledge' and 'evidence'. Again we find the fixity of a paradigm, a stabilisation of knowledge in relation to educational thought, both in how pedagogy is structured and in what it aims towards. The scientific destabilisation found in the likes of Lacan and Kuhn above are refuted in the modelling of education. In this confident affirmation of the model, we witness the attempt to stabilize the symbolic order that bestows its authority of the institutions of education and its subjects.

Even more reductive than the historical emphasis on Piagetian developmental psychology in the classroom (Johnson, 2014) or ZPD (Peim, 2009), the supposed knowledge of recent policy is rooted in linear logics supported by its emphasis on 'memory' (DfE, 2024, p. 13), rooted in cognitive models (pp. 30–35) of the mind as a 'storage system' or 'visuo-spatial sketchpad' (Baddeley, 1992). We can only assume that these are the databases of absolute science that can be thumbed through at will with the appropriate pedagogical methods demanded in the classroom. Through a continuous return to the fully imparted knowledge, the memory bank is established for the student. Though Lacan eventually moved away from the topographical metaphors for his images of mind, learning, knowledge and so forth (something Freud did often), there is an important metaphor of Freud's that exemplifies the contrasting apparatus of memory for psychoanalytic thought. It is found most clearly in Freud's short essay on the magic notepad, mystic writing pad, or magic slate (SE XIX):

> the magic slate [*Wunderblock*], consisting of a thin wax-covered board bound on one edge to, and covered by, a sheet of celluloid, on whose surface one can inscribe and later erase signs. The slate preserves an invisible trace, while also maintaining the prestine virginity of the writing surface. Freud compares this magic slate with the psychic apparatus, which both receives traces without saving them and saves them while at the same time erasing them. The sheet of celluloid represents the preconscious system and the wax-covered board, the unconscious system. (Rudinesco, 1990)

The difference between the *wunderblock* and sketchpads or storage systems where memory can be easily called upon is clear, and evidences the flattening of knowledge as a signifier. The space of knowledge from the psychoanalytic perspective cannot be called upon and drawn upon like opening up a filing cabinet or flipping open a sketchpad. What is left there are only messy traces, sometimes unreadable, and powerfully impactful on the subject that wants (or doesn't want) to access them.

Lacan offers much in the way of thinking through a subject of mastery, a position he refers to as the 'subject who is supposed to know [S.s.S.]' (XI, p. 232) that we discussed in Chap. 2. To reiterate briefly, this subject poses or is positioned as representing a 'corpus of absolute knowledge' (p. 232)—being in effect a non-lacking figure, an imaginary figure that cannot exist, except as a necessary fantasy in our relation with knowledge authority. Lacan of course speaks of S.s.S. as the analyst, someone the patient comes to see believing they know or can come to know what is 'wrong' with the patient. But only the patient knows; the analyst merely helps them uncover that knowledge. As such, there is no S.s.S.; but its illusion is vital in the situation of the psychoanalytic clinic. Unsurprisingly, this idea has been mapped onto teachers in many instances (Felman, 1982; Davis, 1987; Jay, 1987); the teacher as S.s.S. is one who the student believes they can rely on to have knowledge of 'it all', when, as made clear earlier, the subject only partially knows themself, let alone the student's knowledge. It is 'a deceptive position… an illusion, a source of error' (X, p. 59). The order of knowledge that is framed by pedagogy *puts* the teacher in this position, and of course many teachers accept it willingly, but even those who don't still hover there in their relation to the students.

Becoming the S.s.S. is not a recent educational revelation formed by the impetus for subject mastery and knowledge. 'It is the most exacting and intractable imposition that teaching and its institutions put upon an instructor, and the one which must be analyzed and resisted if education is to be something more' (Jay, 1987, p. 785). As such, the positioning of the teacher as S.s.S. in the policy is one that is bound to be replete with anxiety when encountered by the would-be teacher entering the classroom.

> One can tell students the truth, the facts, until the final bell rings, and little of it penetrates, even when students are adept at repeating answers on exams. As long as the student continues to occupy the same position in relation to the information involved—a position in which he or she 'knows' by virtue of identification with the position of the teacher as the subject who knows—then there is no knowing in any productive sense. (Jay, 1987, p. 789).

The way the student will not know, due to reliance on the subject assumed to know, generates demands on the teacher as a subject. Such demands may be fraught with anxiety and discomfort. To paraphrase Lacan, the position in the frame we are made to feel at home in is the place where we find anxiety (X, p. 75). The classroom now unlocked via the gathering of knowledge is of course such a space.

Potential, the *Point-de-Capiton*

To finish this chapter, we might linger on the 'end point' of pedagogy. Here we quote Lacan at length:

> Whether people are civilized or not, enlightened or not, they are capable of the same collective enthusiasms, the same passions. They are always at a level that there is no reason to describe as higher or lower, as affective, passionate, or supposedly intellectual, or developed, as they say ... that should inspire us to take a much more modest view of the possibility of progress in thought. (MT, pp. 104–5)

Over the past decade or so, numerous educational 'reforms' have been taking place in the UK (and elsewhere) as an attempt to, so critics say, narrow the possibilities of teaching.[9] This set of reforms, accompanied by

[9] First there was curriculum and examination reform, with a focus on rigour, final assessments, long-form written exams, and supposedly challenging material. Changes to inspections, the external gaze of the disciplinary Other, came too to discipline the outcomes of schools. Next came an unprecedented intervention into teacher training, with a full 'market

teacher exodus and increase in strikes, highlights a significant split between governmental and practitioner views of education in the UK, and this situation is not remotely particular to the UK. Evidently, the fantasies held by each group clash with one another (as was made clear in Chap. 3). In this clash we most commonly hear complaints of the 'neoliberalisation of learning' invoked even by psychoanalysts (Yates, 2022). Without a doubt, there are difficulties faced by teachers now due to the current political climate, echoed by concerns raised by unions and the everyday teacher in the staffroom. Yet, what this sort of analysis misses is the shared ideal-ego envisioned by so much governmental policy implemented through the reforms (and indeed in countless other historical reforms) and the commonplace teacher. Despite the apparent antithesis, the pedagogical relationship engendered by the teaching stage impels an inevitable end. It is easy to be seduced by the low-hanging fruit in education in terms of ends. Some lament the shift to education as performativity, or as skills trumping knowledge (not just in the classic sense of vocational skills, but also the 'transferable' skills of the fluid workforce). The oft-heard critique is that an education without assessment would allow us to engage in education as a signifier of fullness and plenitude, a non-lacking Other, an education that could just go on and on towards our personal and societal betterment. Though as, Ansgar Allen notes, there is no education without assessment (2014). It is a vital part of its historicity and Symbolic structure: so that we might claim that assessment is precisely what education is for. Without the distinctions confirmed by assessment there is no educational order, no difference between learner and learned. Without

review' of the training providers. Many had their capacity to train teachers stripped away, and those that kept it had to follow a strict framework in their provision. Initial Teacher Education became a 'state franchise with a strong emphasis on fidelity to both mandatory design and content' (Ellis, 2024, p. 1). Retention strategies were implemented too, an attempt to offer more objet a's for early career teachers to ensure the profession remained desirable, mostly in the form of monetisation, extra qualifications, and an emphasis of the moral reward. Thinktanks and research groups (ones that were predominantly in the pockets of the Conservative Government) offered curriculum and pedagogy packages to 'support' teachers, and the narratives around 'lefty' and 'woke' teachers attempting to decolonise, radicalise, Marxify the classroom were rife (these are as much the stuff of fantasy as anything else). Unsurprisingly, an exodus has occurred in the sector, with over '20% of new teachers leav[ing] the profession within their first two years of teaching, and 33% leav[ing] within their first 5 years' (DfE, 2019b, p. 11). Those that remained in the profession balloted to strike, with one major teaching union striking for a number of days for fairer pay, conditions, and support.

assessment there can be no feudal hierarchy that is the grounds for attainment, progress, development—all the favoured features of the educational ideal. Another dimension to this is the almost universal espousal among educators of an (often unconscious) eugenicist belief in intelligence. The everyday discourse of school staffroom (and almost every educational setting you can think of) is replete with references to innate ability. Critiques of assessment as limiting end also neglect a much grander end that is alluded to by radically different camps in educational theory and practice: that there is a path and the end of teaching is that students should be helped to progress to reach their potential. The manner in which the process of progress can occur is open to numerous 'different' pedagogies, curricula, and of course potential is rooted in differing forms of knowledge, skills, and assessments. It is in these different imaginary dimensions of progress and potential that the contemporary political division occurs.

What is most interesting about progress and potential, however, is how they punctuate education. Lacan alludes to the 'order of the signifier' (E, p. 418), that is, the linguistic shape of the Symbolic, and as such includes the structural features of 'grammar' (p. 418). If we retain the Lacanian view of the Symbolic order as grammatical, punctuation gives it pace and shape, like the final word in an exchange between two people. Certain signifiers perform similar functions in education so to arrest its meaning and give it an appearance of solidity and certainty. This is what Lacan calls the *points de capiton* (III, p. 268), the button ties that you might find on a cushion to arrest the fabric. As Lacan says, 'the signifier stops the otherwise endless movement of the signification' (E, p. 303)—a marked complement to Derrida's boundless chains of signification (1976). Even if policy makers and teachers can't agree on what should be taught, how it should be taught, and how it should it be assessed, at least they can agree on something: That education is ultimately about helping students make progress towards their potential. Many of the examples explored in Chap. 3 on teacher fantasies made this point manifestly clear. Though each fantasy differed, at heart they circled around students and their progress towards their brighter futures of fulfilled potential—whether it be the disadvantaged pupils in *Half Nelson,* the troubled prodigy in *Donnie Darko,* the ambitious drummer in *Whiplash,* or the irreverent teens in *Teachers.* Policy documents make regular reference to metonymic signifiers like 'growth', 'development', 'high expectations', and 'achievement'. In the midst of the UK education reforms, the Department for Education released a *Teacher Recruitment and Retention Strategy* (DfE, 2019a) document, similar to many recruitment strategies around the world, that may have been politically unsavoury for many teachers, but still retained the language of teachers who 'inspire children, raising their eyes to a world of possibility and supporting them to fulfil their potential' (p. 4). It is a 'unique' position in 'shaping [students'] future and the future of society' (p. 19). The framework issued to training providers for trainee and earl career teachers decreed that one must hold 'a belief in the academic potential of all pupils' (DfE, 2024, p. 11) and 'promote good progress' (p. 13). Even common parlance in teacher circles, enunciated commonly in books about teaching like *What Great Teachers Do Differently* (Whittaker, 2020), state that one should 'Put students first' and 'Make every decision on what's best for students' (p. 55), but first for what? Best in what sense? It is in such quotidian phrases like these that teachers believe that the goal is the students progressing.

This might seem a strange target for most readers: why should we be concerned about wanting students to do better? An obvious answer would be that any critical approach, be it psychoanalysis, Critical Theory, Marxism, and so forth, should interrogate unthought faiths that exist at every level of social institutions. This is perhaps where the authors' suspicion took hold; there is something fundamentally unsettling, even uncanny, about a universalised mantra for such a mass project as education. But the Lacanian perspective makes this suspicion fundamental to its mode of thought, for you 'will not find in Lacan words like growth' (Webster, 2022, p. 42). Psychoanalysis isn't therapy for Lacan; it isn't getting better, curing, healing, or any other therapeutically loaded terms. What is interesting, as Ecclestone and Hayes (2008) note, is that education takes on similar signifiers in its justification of its place in the Symbolic order, especially in ideas of potential being met for every child.

To allow for potential to be met, other signifiers arise in the signifying chain. 'Inclusion' becomes a buzz word in education and in social services in the early part of this century, touching on the fear of excluded children existing beyond the Symbolic order of progress and normativity. This concern indicates the powerful role of the pedagogical relation in the governance and politics of childhood that occurs significantly at the symbolic level. What's new in the governmental documentation is that 'children' become defined as 'the child', a significant shift of signifier not simply in the unit of address; but also as an Imaginary way of defining the child as a self, a self capable of being administered to (paradoxically perhaps) in terms of self-governance.[10] As global educational policy (UNESCO, 2024) continues to advocate for the agency of the child, seeking to promote (and where necessary to redirect) 'the voice of the child' at the same time they advocate strongly for the juridical and veridical dimensions of governance deeply ingrained in the extensive human technology of the school. Since the inception of the modern school in the second half of the nineteenth century the 'deep grammar' of schooling has been concerned with the formation and refashioning the 'self'. The appeal to 'voice' is presented as inclusive, although voice in the sense used refers, inevitably, to language that, as Lacan would have it, 'speaks me more than I speak it' (E, p. 447).

So the more or less ongoing governmental panics attending exclusions and truancy concern avoiding casualties of social order that we can also interpret as potential failures of the Symbolic order. To be without or outside of the dominant discourse of self-improvement that prevails in the order of education threatens delinquency. The Symbolic order (curriculum/institutional norms of conduct, deportment, orientation) of education is held to have universal reference and address. 'Prevention' of dropouts and of truancy has been an essential component of what Nikolas Rose (1990) has referred to as 'governing the soul'. This work to maintain the universal grip of the Symbolic has been extended through nursery education and various forms of pre-school provision to 'governing the soul' of the community, in practices that labour to ensure that the appropriate educational narrative is being maintained for all. As Rose has also indicated, the emphasis on 'government through community' expressed in extensive government projects such as was the Children's Fund is predicated on addressing 'problem' communities (as locations of social exclusion) at the level of the signifier. In the discourse and the array of practices that attend such governmental concern 'a sector is brought into existence' that is signified as a therapeutic domain to be addressed through 'services' that supplement education. We might characterize this social work as a 'community' talking cure. In the context of what has been defined by Giddens as 'reflexive modernization' we can see the extension of the governmental role of the school into the community through various satellite institutions and practices that are designed to address more recalcitrant individuals, families and communities as symbolic labour. According to Giddens's account of the 'post-traditional order', identity is not inherited

[10] Children addressed by the Children's Fund, for example, as being in danger of exclusion would be given a book entitled 'About Me' in order to rewrite themselves under supervision in line with norms of aspiration that would lead to inclusion.

or static; it becomes a reflexive project—an endeavour to be continuously worked and requiring constant reflection: '… identity is not to be found in behaviour, nor—important though this is—in the reactions of others, but in the capacity to keep a particular narrative going …' (Giddens, 1991, p. 54). Again, it is at the level of the signifier that governing through changes in the Symbolic order are to be managed by 'services'.

In all these examples we see the arresting of the educational process. No matter the calls for 'lifelong learning' heard from typical educational critics, there is a clear desire in each of the examples throughout this chapter to fix an end point to the impossible relationship of pedagogy. This can be as little as learning a new phoneme in a nursery phonics lesson or as major as reinventing the soul of society. The *point de capiton* still positions itself as the closing point of the grammar of education. This ethic of positive, potentially redemptive intervention, state administration—'police' in Foucault's sense—of individuals, families and neighbourhoods occurs through normalizing agencies of social welfare in arrangements that are both more flexible and more oriented towards self-corrective techniques of person and community management. This mode of governmentality requires the mechanisms to distribute the project of self-refashioning as fundamental to prevention and social redemption with education, as orientation to meaning, at the centre. The practices of such symbolic police work are directed to enhance the 'agency' of the 'self' that is required to effect its own transformation and reorientation out of unproductive or negatively productive exclusion. It should not be difficult to see the Lacanian dimension of this in the refashioning of the address and reception of the symbolic order, in the imaginary projection of normative progress, development and achievement both in relation to the untransformed real of social distinctions. Another name for this set of practices might simply be social pedagogy. Of course, there are other forms of pedagogy available. We can hear the readers of the book starting to scream of alternatives, so now we turn to those too.

References

Others

Allen, A. (2014). *Benign Violence: Education in and Beyond the Age of Reason*. Palgrave Macmillan.

Bacon, F. (1902 [1620]). *Novum Organum* (J. Devey, Ed.). P.F. Collier.

Baddeley, A. (1992). Working Memory. *Science, 255*(5044), 556–559.

Barnes, D. (1976). *From Communication to Curriculum*. Penguin.

Barthes, R. (1977). Writers, Intellectuals, Professors. In *Image, Music, Text* (pp. 190–215). Fontana Press.
Bernstein, B. (1975). *Class, Codes and Control: Towards a Theory of Educational Transmission, Volume 3.* Routledge.
Bernstein, B. (1995). *Pedagogy, Symbolic Control and Identity.* Taylor and Francis.
Britton, J. (1970). *Language and Learning.* Penguin.
Britzman, D. (1991). *Practice Makes Practice: A Critical Study of Learning to Teach.* SUNY Press.
Cioran, E.M. (2018 [1975]). *A Short History of Decay.* Penguin Books.
Clarke, M. (2019). Education beyond Reason and Redemption: A Detour Through the Death Drive. *Pedagogy, Culture & Society, 27*(2), 183–197.
Davis, R. C. (1987). Pedagogy, Lacan, and the Freudian Subject. *College English, 49*(7), 749–755.
Derrida, J. (1976). *Of Grammatology* (G. C. Spivak, Trans.). Johns Hopkins University Press.
Derrida, J. (1994). *Specters of Marx: The State of the Debt, the Work of Mourning and the New International.* Routledge.
Derrida, J. (1995). *On the Name* (D. Wood, J. P. Leavy, Jr., & I. McLeod, Trans.). Stanford University.
DfE. (2019a). *Teacher Recruitment and Retention Strategy.* https://www.gov.uk/government/publications/teacher-recruitment-and-retention-strategy
DfE. (2019b). *Character Education Framework.* https://www.gov.uk/government/publications/character-education-framework
DfE. (2024). *Initial Teacher Training and Early Career Framework.* https://assets.publishing.service.gov.uk/media/65b8fa60e9e10a00130310b2/Initial_teacher_training_and_early_career_framework_30_Jan_2024.pdf
Dixon, J. (1967). *Growth through English.* National Association for the Teaching of English.
Dollimore, J., & Sinfield, A. (1985). *Shakespeare.* Manchester University Press.
Drakakis, J. (Ed.). (1985). *Alternative Shakespeares.* Methuen.
Eagleton, T. (1983). *Literary Theory: An Introduction.* University of Minnesota Press.
Ecclestone, K., & Hayes, D. (2008). *The Dangerous Rise of Therapeutic Education.* Routledge.
Edwards, A., & Daniels, H. (2004). Using Sociocultural and Activity Theory in Educational Research. *Educational Review, 56*(2), 107–111.
Ellis, V. (Ed.). (2024). *Teacher Education in Crisis: The State, the Market and the Universities in England.* Bloomsbury Academic.
Ellis, V. , & Childs, A. (2024). Introducing the Crisis: The State, the Market, the Universities and Teacher Education in England. In V. Ellis (Ed.). *Teacher Education in Crisis: The State, the Market and the Universities in England* (pp. 1–26). London,: Bloomsbury Academic. Retrieved May 22, 2025, from http://dx.doi.org/10.5040/9781350399693.ch-1

Engeström, Y. (2003). Activity Theory and Individual and Social Transformation. In Y. Engeström, R. Miettinen, & R.-L. Punamahi (Eds.), *Perspectives on Activity Theory* (pp. 19–38). Cambridge University Press.
Felman, S. (1982). Psychoanalysis and Education: Teaching Terminable and Interminable. *Yale French Studies, 63*, 21–44.
Foucault, M. (1977). *The Archaeology of Knowledge*. Routledge.
Foucault, M. (1991). *Discipline and Punish. The Birth of the Prison*. Penguin.
Giddens, A. (1991). *Modernity and Self-Identity: Self and Society in the Late Modern Age*. Stanford University Press.
Grene, M. (1966). *The Knower and the Known*. University of California Press.
Hochschild, A. (1998). *King Leopold's Ghost: A Story of Greed, Terror, and Heroism in Colonial Africa*. Houghton Mifflin.
Holt, J. (1990). *How Children Fail*. Penguin.
Hordern, J., & Brooks, C. (2023). The Core Content Framework and the 'New Science' of Educational Research. *Oxford Review of Education, 49*(6), 800–818.
Jay, G. S. (1987). The Subject of Pedagogy: Lessons in Psychoanalysis and Politics. *College English, 49*(7), 785–800.
Johnson, T. R. (2014). *The Other Side of Pedagogy: Lacan's Four Discourses and the Development of the Student Writer*. SUNY Press.
Kristeva, J. (1984). *Revolution in Poetic Language*. Columbia University Press.
Kuhn, T. (1970). *The Structure of Scientific Revolutions*. Chicago University Press.
Latour, B. (1988). *Science in Action*. Harvard University Press.
Lyotard, J. F. (1979). *The Postmodern Condition: A Report on Knowledge*. Manchester University Press.
McGowan, T. (2013). *Enjoying What We Don't Have: The Political Project of Psychoanalysis*. University of Nebraska Press.
Miller, J-A. (2006). The Symptom: Knowledge, Meaning and the Real. *The Symptom*, 7.
Moran, D. (2000). *Introduction to Phenomenology*. Routledge.
Peim, N. (2009). Activity Theory and Ontology. *Educational Review, 61*(2), 167–180.
Peim, N. (2018). *Thinking in Education Research*. Bloomsbury.
Rose, N. S. (1990). *Governing the Soul: The Shaping of the Private Self*. Routledge.
Rudinesco, E. (1990). *Lacan and Derrida in the History of Psychoanalysis*. Lecture Held October 15, 1990, at Columbia University in New York. Available in *European Journal of Psychoanalysis*, 2, Fall 1995–Winter 1996.
Stock, N. (2024). Classroom Architecture and the Gaze. Beyond the Panopticon. *Discourse: Studies in the Cultural Politics of Education, 45*(4), 521–535.

UNESCO. (2024). *Global Education Monitoring Report, 2024/5, Leadership in Education: Lead for Learning*. https://unesdoc.unesco.org/ark:/48223/pf0000391406.locale=en
Vygotsky, L. S. (1978). *Mind in Society: The Development of Higher Psychological Processes*. Harvard University Press.
Watts, J. (Ed.). (1977). *The Countesthorpe Experience*. Allen and Unwin.
Webster, J. (2022). *Disorganization and Sex*. Divided.
Whittaker, T. (2020). *What Great Teachers Do Differently: Nineteen Things That Matter Most* (3rd ed.). Routledge.
Yates, C. (2022). The Tensions of Teaching Psychoanalysis in the Neoliberal University. *New Associations*, 38.

CHAPTER 5

The Impossibility of Pedagogical Alternatives

Abstract This chapter addresses the idea of critical pedagogy that so much academic educational commentary depends on: the idea of another, more educational mode of education. Here we reconsider liberatory pedagogy in the likes of Freire, Giroux, Aronowitz and Ranciere through the lens of Lacanian intersubjective modelling. We produce a critique of 'critical pedagogy' including ideas associated with Apple and Biesta. The idea of the child in modernity is set alongside 'destructive plasticity' leading into an account of the Lacanian death drive, realigning all ideas of liberatory pedagogy with desire. A thorough account of the impossibility of the pedagogic relation is provided, and then aligned with the idea of a 'pedagogized society'.

Keywords Critical pedagogy • Radical pedagogy • Liberatory pedagogy • Death drive • Desire • Phallus • Lack • Pedagogical relationship • Plasticity • Consciousness raising • Anti-pedagogy

...there is such a thing as a teacher's desire.
—(Jacques Lacan, Seminar X, p. 172)

© The Author(s), under exclusive license to Springer Nature Switzerland AG 2025

N. Stock, N. Peim, *The Lacanian Teacher*, The Palgrave Lacan Series, https://doi.org/10.1007/978-3-031-93018-8_5

Liberatory Pedagogy

Ivan Illich, radical thinker of deschooling, once said to Paulo Freire, another radical educational thinker, that his methods of pedagogy were a 'kind of historico-cultural, political psychoanalysis' (in Freire, 2014, p. 60). In fact, in Freire's later reflective work, he refers to the students of his classroom as 'educands', a clear reformulation of the 'analysand' of the psychoanalytic clinic—the patient on the couch. One would think, therefore, that this sort of pedagogy offers a 'way out' of the scenes we have examined in the previous chapter: the structure of pedagogy as it habitually plays out in the classroom of the school or in the university. The importance of mundane pedagogy lies in the relationships to students and to knowledge that the vast majority of teachers are Symbolically inscribed into. We recognise that there are claims made for alternative forms and models of pedagogy that many would say run contrary to our analysis, and even, like Illich said, make psychoanalytic strides in pedagogical restructuration. This is the case in one respect, as in the more radical and liberatory forms of pedagogy that get promoted there is a different relationship projected between teacher and student. Moreover, in these cases we often find knowledge is replaced by other signifiers of lack like 'consciousness' or 'freedom' as being the pedagogic desiderata—a substitution, or perhaps deferral, of the *objet a* in the fundamental fantasy of the educator. What we contend, however, is that so-called alternative pedagogies share the same Symbolic space and the same problems that we have uncovered via Lacan in dominant forms of pedagogy, especially when read alongside the work of Julie Reshe (2017, 2023).

One might notice that the description of pedagogy that we detailed throughout Chap. 4 is an echo of Freire's reportedly 'radical' critique of education found in his landmark text *Pedagogy of the Oppressed*. Indeed, as authors we have regularly faced contestation from audience members at conferences that our analysis of education pertains to what Freire calls the 'banking concept' (1993, p. 45) of pedagogy, and that there are radical alternatives available that deflate our claims. The signifiers of 'conscientização' (1993, p. 41; something akin to critical consciousness) and 'Hope, especially' (2014, p. 41) become the *objet a* of the pedagogical relationship rather than something more epistemological as we discussed in the previous chapter. In some of these instances at conferences, Freire is invoked as a master signifier, a trump card that forecloses critique of the idea of a pure or proper education. Nevertheless, we will look more closely at the ideas of Freire and some of his descendants to show why we believe this to be a misguided argument.

Freire's contention is that dominant forms of pedagogy are based on three presuppositions:

> a) the teacher teaches and the students are taught; (b) the teacher knows everything and the students know nothing; (c) the teacher thinks and the students are thought about… (1993, p. 46)

This model, Freire claims, sustains oppression thus foreclosing critical consciousness in the student, neatly mirroring the pedagogy of right-wing and authoritarian education fostered and growing in many schools and universities at the current moment (Hursh, 2018; Robertson & Nestore, 2021; Salajan & Jules, 2024). At the heart of Freire's critique is the notion that students are treated as empty vessels to be filled—a constitution of lack from the oppressor that is to be, the educator says, remedied by education. This is a gifting of a signifier of lack from one to the other, done graciously or oppressively, substantiating the master as the S.s.S. To repeat, it is at this moment that the writers of this book often face much opposition, as Freire and the various descendants of critical pedagogy have claimed to move beyond 'banking' in education. In doing so, they claim to have escaped from the authoritarian jouissance of non-lack at play in the conventional classroom. However, we find that this representation of critical pedagogy is an integral aspect of the educational Imaginary, and constitutes another logic essential in perpetuating its Symbolic order. The pedagogical relationship does not exist, whether critical or not. It is important to also state here, as we have done in Chap. 3, that in no way do we believe this book offers anything like an escape or an outside from education. The presentation of our fantasies hopefully makes this clear, and indeed the final chapter will offer only a mode of reorienting enjoyment *in* the classroom space, not somehow going beyond or outside of it.

Working through Freire's counter-pedagogical model, we might initially find resonance between his and Lacan's claims as Illich did. It seems Freire aims towards a situation that mirrors Lacan's Symbolic/Real dimensions, where 'the Subject recognize himself in the object (the coded concrete existential situation) and recognizes the object as a situation in which he finds himself, together with other Subjects' (Freire, 1993, p. 78). Freire's version is that the subject, previously denied their full subjecthood and treated merely as object, needs to be led to recognise that their objectness is merely the situation (Symbolic space) they are in, not their fundamental state of being. The educator is vital in the task of allowing them to see this, so to realise their full subjectivity. This is a crucial move in enabling the apprehension of what Freire takes as reality, so to allow the subjects of his pedagogy to critically intervene. But the conceptions of subjects, relations, and pedagogy require further consideration from the Lacanian perspective, especially in a process that is predicated on the interplay of lack and pursuit of what is lacked. Clearly, Freire retains the idea that the subject can be made a 'whole self' (2014, p. 41). What we have shown in the previous chapters, particularly in Chap. 2, is that the Lacanian subject is a subject *of* lack. They are always-already castrated, unable to fully realise their desire, impotently grasping for recognition. This slightly more (some might say) dismal view of the subject already puts a bump in the road of Freire's method. It implies that no model of education could remedy this primordial lack (though some perhaps might allow us to interrogate it better). The student of critical pedagogy on the path to wholeness is only going to be met with the anxiety of impossibility in becoming this whole self.

We also find in Freire, despite the attempt to 'resolve the teacher-student contradiction' (1993, p. 48) by dethroning the position of the teacher, the lingering trace of the belief in the liberatory power of the signifier of lack. Freire's logic still can't rid the pedagogic scene of the teacher figure who stands in a privileged relation to the order of knowledge that cannot be revealed wholesale in the 'classroom'. What Freire, and much 'progressive', liberal and liberating pedagogy, seems to want to do is to shift the order of knowledge from the externally ensconced archive with its global apparatus of institutions and practices, to the determination of the self. The Freirean pedagogue wants to enable the Freirean student to empower their own potential in a mutually engaging process. As he says,

> any political and educational plans have failed because their authors designed them according to their own personal views of reality, never once taking into account (except as mere objects of their actions) *the men-in-a-situation* to whom their program was ostensibly directed. (1993, p. 67)

What he proposes is a teacher as a subject free from the ego-ideal, disentangled from the gaze, fantasy free. We know this position is an impossible one to occupy; we remain subjects constituted by these different elements. Indeed, Freire emphasises the dialogic aspects of his method, a 'problem-posing method—dialogical par excellence (1993, p. 82). It 'must not be transformed into a noncommittal "chewing the fat" to the random rhythm of whatever happens to be transpiring between teacher and educands' (2014, p. 123). In this sense, it maintains a *relation* between teacher and student, and as there still has to be a pedagogy and a pedagogue for this process to occur, we still find traces of the differential relation. In both liberatory and typical forms of pedagogy, there must be a teaching stage that in relation to the signifier of lack in the designation of Other. There has to be a Freire (or similar), after all, in the critical pedagogical relationship to allow the forum to take place. They act as the master signifier of the relationship, that which compels the educational act to begin whilst also receding into the background might be a form of veiling. This 'veil' (E, p. 579) of the figure, Lacan suggests, is actually imbued with further strength and mystery. Not least we can see this in the *way* figures like Freire are invoked as some sort of pedagogical master.

Still, the pedagogue who disavows their position as master (whilst still upholding the other as lacking in critical consciousness) invests in identification of the Other as 'Child'—a master signifier of its own with a complex ontological structure, driving much of educational activity (or passivity). As Reshe notes,

> Thinkers who contributed to the development of the modern concept of child perceived children not just as those who have to be educated by educators, but also simultaneously as those who are themselves educable: who are moldable by their nature. (2017, p. 169)

This moldability positions the Child as inherently educable, the one that demands education—under an imperative that drives the teacher to educate. It is interesting that many teachers of course note the failure of this demand, something that often realigns them with one of the perverse fantasies of education such as the masochist up all night marking or the sadist doling out discipline. Britzman gives further weight to this claim (1991, p. 179). One teacher she interviews clearly finds the demand lacking from his students but looks for it in training teachers, whom he perceives to have an instant and tangible impact on; when we think the educable is absent, we look for it elsewhere. It is no coincidence that the rise of the schooled society coincides, in the west at least, with the invention of childhood (Aries, 1962; Coveney, 1967; Cunningham, 2005). National curricula indicate something of the intense onto-politics invested in this highly developed form of age-stratification.

Many other unconscious elements permeate the putative pedagogic relation, of course, but the gifting of the signifier of lack is Symbolic only. This enjoyment that so many teachers likely find themselves amidst is both one of political concern if we are to believe Freire, and one without any real substance. As Britzman asks, 'might this subject [of the teacher] be inseparable from the anticipations, wishes, ideas, phantasies, and beliefs held for education?' (2015, p. 12) rather than the relation they believe to be taking place, or *wishes* was taking place? Does the moment that even the idealised educational forum of critical pedagogy actually pertain to the pure educational goal that has been set, or does it really trade in the Real—no matter what form it takes? Indeed, might we even say that such a belief in 'the' pedagogical relation is an attempt to hide the castration of the subject of the teacher, to maintain the belief that they hold the signifier of lack, the knowledge and the *nous*, that can be imparted to the Other? In this fantasy, the non-lacking dimension is maintained by the projection of the other as recipient of 'empowerment'.

One might think that this shift in perspective of knowledge has been addressed by Jacques Ranciere in *The Ignorant Schoolmaster* (1991), where the 'hero', Jacatot, does not instruct the students, but rather leaves them to search for and create the knowledge themselves. Jacatot doesn't go home and rethink his career path, though. Somehow, he must be on or in the scene. There is something alluring in this endlessly repeated example of the progressive model, the Countesthorpe ethic, we might call it, that seems to liberate the teacher from the police function, that relies on a withdrawal of that function.[1] That very withdrawal indicates its more powerful inscription in the collective imaginary. The symbolic order of the institution is functioning no less powerfully for being internalised and acceded to by the self-directing pupils/students. And, as Catherine Malabou points out, *The Ignorant Schoolmaster* positions Jacatot as the authoritative witness, the one who reveals and sustains the key idea that

[1] Countesthorpe College was a custom built (1970) progressive state school (14–19) in Leicestershire that was run as a democracy and that gained both fame and notoriety as a new model school where students would set their own timetable and manage their own learning (Watts, 1977).

equality of intelligence must be a given. It is therefore, as she puts it, 'archic' as opposed to being anarchic (Malabou, 2023, p. 207); it is another veiling of the mysterious educational figure, a different configuration of the Other as 'witness' (E, p. 684).

Destructive Pedagogy

To repeat then, if we are not to seek knowledge, what follows for pedagogy? Here it seems easy to fall in the trap laid by the educational Symbolic order, one that we as authors have encountered too many times to mention in our encounter with critical educational theorists. This trap is that we should—eschewing the pursuit of knowledge—follow the teachings of Freire and the school of critical pedagogy to raise the consciousness of oppressed subjects to allow them to act as agents in their liberation. Indeed, two of Freire's acolytes, Henry Giroux and Stanley Aronowitz, unknowingly alert us to other issues from the Lacanian perspective. Both Giroux (2010) and Aronowitz (1998, 2008, 2009) emphasise a central function of critical pedagogy as its acculturation of agency in the student. This agency is to allow the student to seek their own path, to challenge the dominant paradigms of oppression they find themselves within: an honourable endeavour, of course. But Lacan's theory of the subject complicates the very agency they aim towards, posing a fatal wound to the gospel, goals and methods of critical pedagogy. If we take Aronowitz's claim, that critical pedagogy is 'to encourage human agency, not mould it in the manner of Pygmalion' (1998, pp. 10–11), we are left to ponder the mode of formation, or subjectivation, being proposed. Aronowitz's opposition to moulding looks like another attempt to fade out the figure of the educator, insinuating a flattened classroom where students are only encouraged, nurtured or fostered by the teacher, rather than taught. Similarly, Michael Apple's espousal of critical education in the face of the occupation of education by governmental forces of instrumentalism, echoes Gert Biesta's theological faith in education as absolutely central to what is properly human (Apple, 2006; Biesta, 2006). Both promote the idea of an education proper but neglect to acknowledge the logic of the pedagogical scene. What agency can the educator possibly hope to prompt, an educator that must still (oddly perhaps) be present, if they are not the master of their own agency, even master of their own house to paraphrase Freud? Teacher agency is always already challenged by 'what Lacan would consider to be the impenetrable kernel of the Real that lies at the core of our being, such that 'some parts of ourselves will always remain enigmatic and indecipherable ... we are never fully transparent to ourselves or to others' (Clarke & Kennedy, 2024, p. 11). The pedagogic scene as envisaged by Aronowitz, Giroux, Apple and others is abstracted from the institution that gives it occasion for being. And a significant dimension of that institution—that lends its authority and its aura to the educator—is not just the school but the Symbolic order that is always already loaded with meaning and intention beyond the reach and control of its subjects.

Such a view is once again invested in the position of the Child mentioned previously. Despite the claim that the student can be taught and become anything, it disguises the child's plasticity for flexibility (Malabou, 2010). As Reshe asserts:

> In terms of flexibility, a child is perceived as an obedient passive material that needs to be formed. Whereas in terms of plasticity, she is perceived as actively involved in her own formation: her learning is understood as her own achievement and as a result of her being active. (2017, p. 169)

Plasticity, the capacity to both be formed and annihilate form, is foreclosed by the commonsense perceptions of knowledge as a developmental progression—something Freire alerted us to in his opposition to the banking model. But we, and indeed Reshe, are wary of subscribing to the adoption of plasticity simply as a synonym for critical pedagogy, another form of enjoyment of non-lack that is 'also fraught with the danger of slipping into an understanding of students as flexible' (p. 170), that is, docile vessels. Ultimately, any form of pedagogy as we have described it here invested in transmission and transformation, whether that be technical, liberatory, or of the self, positions the teacher as 'an adult ... understood as someone who knows what kind of information should be kept from a child and someone who possesses knowledge that has to be conveyed to the child through the process of education' (p. 174). While Reshe is drawn to Catherine Malabou's ontological principal of plasticity, she chooses to focus especially on Malabou's later articulation of 'destructive plasticity' (2010, 2012; a fascinating extension to her ontological challenge to Derrida that draws attention to the existence of 'the unhealably wounded', 'the unfixable' ... 'changed beyond recognition' 'no longer themselves' they exist, wounded beyond cure...') challenging conventional thinking and rethinkings of identity. It is important for both Malabou and Reshe, reading Malabou, that the idea of 'destructive plasticity' tracks back into modern biological sciences to understand processes of life and growth. One interesting dimension of this is that destructive plasticity cannot be read as life expressing its will to power against death, inviting us to reconsider fundamental principles of life.

For Reshe 'destructive plasticity' is 'my favourite concept ever' (2023, p. 48). Reshe acknowledges Malabou's recognition of the tragic in this realization that refuses, at the ontological level, the therapeutic idea. She wants to expand Malabou's 'destructive plasticity' into 'a more general negative anthropological model' (p. 19) and to question Malabou's implicit distinction between 'the alive living' (p. 20) and 'the living dead' (p. 4): to redefine life as a form of death: 'Essentially we are all dead on arrival' suffering 'the illusion of being alive' as we 'imitate life' (p. 21). Her argument here is very sophisticated. She draws on Freud's[2] 'death-drive'—a turn in Freud's thinking, but also perhaps a turn in thinking itself—that has to acknowledge the destructive forces that co-exist with erotic, productive impulses. But she complains that Freud 'ultimately succumbs to the temptation of meaning': accusing Lacan also—and falsely, we think—that he 'didn't capture a properly tragic dimension of life' she sees in 'the impossibility of integration' (p. 25). Reshe prefers the dark but beautifully succinct thinking of Peter Wessel Zappfe, author of 'The Last Messiah' (1933) who eschews all taint of the therapeutic positive and sees the human as an evolutionary error like the mousse whose antlers make effective living impossible. She embraces and co-opts Malabou's destructive plasticity as a 'radical enhancement of Freud's concept of the death drive' suggesting an 'alterity with no remedy' at work in the human psyche (p. 26). For Lacan himself, the death drive 'opens a strain of a totally different nature' (XVI, p. 95), a radical alterity indeed that resists integration into the neat symbolic order of education or the world more broadly.

To confirm the ontological credentials of her pessimism, Reshe (like Malabou's delving into biological science for a new interpretation of the 'meaning of life') draws on contemporary biological thinking. Reshe writes that in neurology 'destructive processes' have been understood teleologically in terms of a reductive dialectic (generation/

[2] It should also be noted that she draws heavily on the erased thought of Sabina Spierlrein, who is credited with discovering the death drive in 1912, years before Freud's *Beyond the Pleasure Principle*.

destruction—synthesis/higher formation). They must now be understood in terms of plasticity as an inherently negative process: 'What we call healing within a positive framework should rather be seen as a modification within the register of the negative' (2023, p. 28). Again, referring back to Malabou, Reshe goes on to elaborate her promotion of the anti-teleological, anti-theological against 'primarily progressive generative processes' in relation to brain development. Reshe declares the 'tragic essence' of the brain's work' that its activity is essentially 'nothing else but extended suicide' structured by 'suicidal vulnerability' (p. 29). From cell biology Reshe adopts the term 'apoptosis'—cell death conceived of as a suicide-like activity, so there is 'neuronal sacrifice' essential to the development of mental structures. In addition, she cites Dalanda on DNA: claiming that as embryo DNA has no blueprint, genes simply channel and constrain with no positive teleology built in (p. 30).

Growth occurs epigenetically through learning: but Reshe is quick to point out that according to cell biologists Chialvo and Bak (p. 33) all learning occurs essentially by moving through mistakes, so that 'the environment acts as a critic rather than a teacher' and learning is predicated on 'negative feedback'. Learning is 'a negative process': 'to fail is not optional' … 'it is the very negative core of learning' (p. 34). She adds that 'The switch of perspective articulated by Chialvo and Bak suggests 'the extension of the concept of destructive plasticity to designate plasticity as such' (p. 34). Here she is referring to brain plasticity but it feels like she wants destructive plasticity to displace plasticity as the ontological principle. This aligns with Reshe's very interesting reclaiming of the 'death drive' not, as with Freud, as a counter-current to life-affirming 'eros'; but (as with Sabine Spielrein whose idea predates Freud's) the essence of the drive in general. In this way she can explain the contemporary crisis of ecological catastrophe and its persistent disavowal.[3] This disavowal is essential. In tracing its place in education, we might see how the pedagogical relationship of any kind imagined as holding the kernel of liberation, even if that must be obtained through a full reorientation of the educator as in Freire and his followers, is something that attempts to

[3] In 'The Changing Child' (2017) Reshe suggests that the necessary 'change of perspective' in epigenetically oriented plasticity changes the ontological status of childhood requiring the reshaping of concept of education, 'unveiling it as a purposeless process without an end.'

disavow the death drive as explored in Reshe's work. The path of pedagogy towards an eventual self-liberation cannot be imagined in this Freudo-Reshean perspective.

Pedagogies of Desire

Like Illich, others have explored the links between pedagogy (especially as consciousness raising) and psychoanalysis—including of the Lacanian variety. A compelling example is the street education initiative *Projeto Axe* in Salvador, Brazil, where Freirean principles were put into practice in various ways. They claimed to be pursuing a pedagogy of desire, inspired by Lacan, to avoid 'the development of resistance in the students by understanding the relationship between the symbolic and the real' (Rossatto, 2002, p. 165). Here we find that the educator is now imbued with even stronger powers than the typical teacher, now able to not only teach and raise consciousness, but also act as a psychoanalyst themselves. They are able to teach students how they can parse the Symbolic and Real, though of course this offers a fundamental misreading of Lacan where the Real can be grasped as reality.

Daniel Cho (2009) offers further Lacanian critique of critical pedagogy by recognising the repression of the *unconscious* at play in *consciousness* raising activities. Instead of just trying to strengthen consciousness, Cho calls for a space for the repressed oppression of the subjects in the pedagogical mode to play out through the mode of transference with an Other. Put differently, the educator comes to unconsciously occupy the position of, say, parent or dictator for the student, so the student can enact their unconscious repressions on the educator. This is something that will happen in education spaces regardless, after all being spaces of transference as we discuss at the end of this chapter. As such, though Cho underscored some of the flaws of critical pedagogy, there is a clear intention to retain the salvific, and thus phantasmatic, dimension of pedagogy: 'One must make an ethical decision to become the subject of the transference in order to achieve the ends of social justice' (p. 108). Despite the utilisation of some psychoanalytic and indeed Lacanian concepts, the ethical dimension of teaching in its Imaginary relation with social justice is asserted once more.

Examples of modifications to the thinking of pedagogy are echoed in other psychoanalytic works on education, each expressing differing degrees of negativity. Shoshona Felman's famous paper, from which the epigram of this chapter is taken, is clear to retain the concept of pedagogy in psychoanalytic thinking. She claims that we should resist the 'desire to escape the pedagogical imperative: a desire—whether possible or impossible—to do away with pedagogy altogether' (1982, p. 23), a desire that the authors of this book hold onto, but also recognise its impossibility. Deborah Britzman claims that pedagogy is the result of anxiety—the anxiety of students not being able to do anything (or do anything without the teacher in the room): 'pedagogy emerges from anxiety over losing the topic and being left only with what is impossible for the students' (p. 56). Tamara Bibby's psychoanalytic account of teaching (2011, pp. 23–124) is less critical, still relying heavily on the necessity of the pedagogical relationship and expounding its foundational structure for learning. Felman, Britzman and Bibby, although to different degrees, retain the Symbolic function of education found in much research that we discussed in Chap. 1: it is a system that needs refinement to enable the learning of all; any complications are mere glitches, accidental intrusions of the Real, rather than our position: that the very nature of the Symbolic order of education and its most common Imaginary manifestation pedagogy are impossible.

Nevertheless, many interventions into pedagogy Felman makes are worth consideration. Felman raises the pedagogy of both Freud and Lacan, making a strong objection to Freud being defined as 'The Anti-Pedagogue', noting how this

> fails to see that every true pedagogue is in effect an anti-pedagogue, not just because every pedagogy has historically emerged as a critique of pedagogy … but because, in one way or another, every pedagogy stems from its confrontation with the impossibility of teaching. (1982, p. 24)

Or, more succinctly, 'an anti-pedagogue is *the* pedagogue par excellence' (p. 24). Felman's dialectical reversal, that those who most strongly contest pedagogy, acknowledging the impossibility of teaching because of the impossibility of knowledge transmission and knowing the Other, subjectivates the pedagogue, the true pedagogue. We must confront two things with Felman here: firstly, an idealism that a true pedagogue and a false pedagogue are plausible, and, secondly, we also find in this a preoccupation with a fantasmatic image of the educator. For, though Felman might bring pedagogy into contention, her upholding of the pedagogue (the true pedagogue as anti-pedagogue) implies education is still the *conditio sine qua non* of our human experience. Is a non-pedagogue only the policeman who refuses to carry a gun? A 'knowledge guru' free from the constraints of the school? Such a signifier implies a teaching and being-a-teacher independent of any institutional context, something that is difficult to reconcile in the face of the staging of teaching as we have described it.

> For teaching to be realized, for knowledge to be learnt, the position of alterity is therefore indispensable: knowledge is what is already there, but always in the Other. Knowledge, in other words, is not a substance but a structural dynamic: it is not contained by any individual but comes about out of the mutual apprenticeship between two partially unconscious speeches which both say more than they know. Dialogue is thus the radical condition of learning and of knowledge, the analytically constitutive condition through which ignorance becomes structurally informative; knowledge is essentially, irreducibly dialogic. (p. 33)

What we posit here then is a doubling—both an acceptance of the impossibility of pedagogy, and a refutation of the implicit dialectical reversal that this gives space for the pedagogue *par excellence*. Like Lacan, the pedagogue must remain present, effaced, without direction—especially the direction of the educational big Other. It is this doubling that we will explore in the final chapter, a doubling that retains the possibility of jouissance without the function of the signifier of lack reigning in the classroom.

There's No Such Thing as a Pedagogical Relationship

Thus far, we have imagined the typical classroom teacher and the critical pedagogue as pedagogical operators who necessarily sustain the signifier of lack in their educational endeavours. This position, we have started to proffer, is one that has its own form of enjoyment. We can take this further if we follow Lacan's later work on sexual relationships. Lacan presents an enigmatic diagram in Seminar XX referred to now as the graph of sexuation. We will not give a full exegesis of this graph (see Copjec, 2015 for an excellent one), but we extract from it some key explorations of the sexed relationship that are notably relevant to the pedagogical relationship. Lacan offers us a map for examining how we are situated in Imaginary identifications within a Symbolic structure. It is a *descriptive* graph, not a proscriptive or essentialist one, that attempts to describe the modes through which a patriarchal division of sex and gender occurs in the world. This 'ordering' of the 'normative concept of genital heterosexuality' (Rose, 1985, p. 35) is a process Lacan calls sexuation. It also refers to the phallus and the sexed body, but we must make clear that we are not referring exactly to sexuation or the phallus here. Instead, we take these ideas from Lacan as symbols for describing the pedagogical relationship as it often plays out in relation to signifiers of lack, such as knowledge, consciousness, hope, and so forth. Ultimately, it is worth considering this graph for Lacan's provocative claim 'there's no such thing as a sexual relationship' (XX, p. 12)—opening the possibility of an impossibility of all types of relationships.

The graph of sexuation positions 'men' and 'women' in relation to the signifier of lack (XX, p. 7): men are designated as such and then thrown into a Symbolic world that impels them to believe they are figures that have the potential to be non-lacking—a status that Lacan makes clear is that of a 'fraud' (Rose, 1985, p. 40). Man is situated as desiring the signifier of lack, but of course never obtains it as the subject remains always wounded and lacking. Lacan then proposes that there is man and the other—anything that is not man and has no pretence that they hold the signifier of lack (XX, p. 7). The subject and its other are designated by this orientation to lack, this 'idea of self-completion through another' (Rose, 1985, p. 36)—and we can start to map the pedagogical relationship here. The signifier of absolute knowledge, mastery, liberation, freedom, or at heart, education, is grasped at by the educator in their desire to enact the pedagogical relationship and agreed as lacking in the student as the other.

In the graph, the lacking other, for us the student, is also further designated by this relationship in a position of conscious lack (p. 7) that can be cured. The logic goes that the figure who believes they *can* obtain the signifier of lack can give it to the other, so to cure their lack. Filling gaps (p. 8) thus become the terrain of jouissance (even the very lack of the supposed holder of the signifier of lack). The student who has a knowledge gap to be filled, an empty depository or bucket, is designated for the relation. The figure who claims, impossibly, to hold the signifier of lack, finds jouissance in being seen as the figure who holds it. None more so than the realm of government, action hero, or of course classroom teacher, armed with disciplinary intent and a head full of knowledge.

The 'relationship cannot be written' (p. 35), and it is writing, the effect of the signifier, that precludes the relationship. In this writing, '"man" and "woman" are mere signifiers that are altogether related to the "curcurrent" use of language' (p. 35). It is only in their designation as man and woman, or as any signifier of difference, that the relationship is expected to be a tessellation of lacking and non-lacking that has no grounding in the Real. So too do the signifiers 'teacher' and 'student', a similar 'tessellatory' relationship. In terms of 'jouissance', this is the enjoyment that is to be found in the belief that one possesses and uses the signifier of lack. As we have said in the previous sections, many teachers might be experiencing this mode of jouissance in the way they teach others, putting knowledge into the heads of students or allowing them to become whole through other means. We find an apposite claim in Seminar VIII where Lacan notes that in the act of the subject's relation to an other is an attempt to 'bring [the other] jouissance ... to perfect him' (VIII, p. 144). The jouissance of the relation is one of completion—a powerful educational myth, even and especially in critical approaches to pedagogy where the student does this independently after an initial pedagogical encounter with the teacher.

None of this is to say, of course, that *nothing* Real takes place in the pedagogical relationship. In fact, part of the thrust of this book is that the relationship is far more interesting than the educational enframing gives it credit for. However, what we find in this relationship is not the actuality of the taking hold of the signifier of lack, but rather the process of transference (Pagès, 2025). First discovered by Freud (SE XII), transference is the unconscious effect of any relationship in which signifiers are exchanged. As we have said previously in this book, the classroom is a space dominated by signifiers. It is primarily a talking space, even in the lecture hall where only the teacher talks. The exchange of signifiers, 'communication' as we most commonly call it, is central to teaching. Most people, especially teachers, believe that communication is 'a direct circuit from speaker to listener' (Webster, 2022, p. 70)—a fantasy of the pedagogical relationship in its Real tessellation. From the psychoanalytic perspective, to speak is a terrifying thing, as it always carries a trace of the unconscious. Enunciation is replete with anxiety and intimacy (p. 69), with the former perhaps being the dominant affect for students in the classroom or teachers with new class. If I open my mouth, how can I know that Other will hear what I meant? We are, after all, 'not in control of our message' (p. 69).

But in terms of pedagogy, what we must emphasise is that for Lacan 'speaking and listening is the engine of transference, nothing more' (p. 70). Put differently, when the teacher speaks to the student and the student listens, or the reverse takes place, there is certainly an exchange of signifiers taking place. But this exchange is unconscious. To quote Britzman at length:

> The transference does not stop at the psychoanalyst's door. It knocks about in pedagogical relations, theories of learning, viewpoints, and arguments. It rattles our learning constructs, procedures, and curricular goals. It binds our misperceptions and confuses reality and phantasy. In the classroom, too, the teacher as character—her passion, knowledge, and authority, and her ignorance, mistakes, and indifference—is oddly familiar and so animates the student and teacher's transference of love and hate onto the presence of pedagogy. Yes, the transference has a different flavor in the classroom, though the problem of unwilling recognition—the emotional situation of not wanting to know anything about that—leaves indigestion, even as we try to relieve it with the antacid of pedagogy that we must also admit is hard to swallow. Pedagogy must gamble with new and old knowledge and the vulnerabilities, hardships, and hurt feelings that the transference conveys and that the emotional situation of teaching and learning also stirs. (Britzman, 2015, p. 34)

And thus, the lesson we think is being taught is neither being thought nor being taught. This is the 'flavour' that Britzman highlights, as there is a whole set of educational fantasies, positions and Symbolic demands taking place in it and through it that do not occur elsewhere—exactly the sorts of things we have explored in the book up to this point.

What we finish with, then, is that this relationship is still worth retaining and reimagining, even if it is not for the purpose of pedagogy. The space of the classroom that we have examined in much detail renders subjects in an interesting relationship with one another than does not and cannot aim towards any attenuation of lack or sense of completion, but nevertheless has interesting unconscious desires being enacted that we examine in the final chapter. We do wonder whether, for example, acknowledging lack as fundamental to the subject might have some sort of 'liberating' effect, but not in the sense of liberating through the acquisition of a signifier of lack. That is, something like knowledge as power, or a sense of true sight of the subject's position in the order in which they reside, so that (oppressed) students might finally see and understand the conditions of their oppression, all the better to address them. Acknowledging the condition of lack in, say, the sense of Julie Reshe's (2023) recent work offers a more modest accommodation, eschewing the promise of liberation through knowledge. The liberating gospel (the 'good news') Reshe proposes is more attuned to a tragic sensibility: life is suffering; you can't be happy/complete, so your condition of lack is inherent. Positively, we can be alone together: not in some ideal community that is both exclusive and excluding but in communion. Reshe's thinking is steeped in powerful exponents of a tragic conception. Her major statement, *Negative Psychoanalysis for the Living Dead: Philosophical Pessimism and the Death Drive*, unites psychoanalysis with a philosophy of pessimism. The dedication of the book is: 'To my daughter, Zoe, who makes my death worth living' (2023, dedication). Reshe wants to offer, quite seriously, a negative alternative to what she calls contemporary 'therapeutic culture', not unlike what we have outlined in the pedagogical culture.

We will therefore work with some of these ideas but emphasise the Lacanian aspects. Reshe promotes a 'depressive realist perspective' claiming that negative psychoanalysis declares the 'disaster of human existence' as against positive 'escapist positions' (p. vii). Trauma is fundamental: veiled or not: 'We ourselves are nothing else but the work of trauma' (p. 20). Rather than seeking to diagnose the ailing and the wounded as special cases, she asks: 'what if the whole world' 'is terminally sick with the same condition' (p. 3)? She cites Philip Rieff who identifies the 'omnipresent psychologization of society' subject to the therapeutic turn seeking to invite cure or preferably 'self-cure' as offering false and misleading hope always destined for disappointment (p. 5). Similarly, we might find the Bernsteinian 'pedagogized society' that privileges education as the proper expression of the truly human, that ends up positioning all in a condition of remediable lack (of knowledge, of critical consciousness), as improperly holding education as the source of both individual and collective salvation, and similarly doomed to disappointment.

References

Others

Apple, M. (2006). *Educating the Right Way*. Routledge.

Aries, P. (1962). *Centuries of Childhood: A Social History of Family Life*. Jonathan Cape.

Aronowitz, S. (1998). *Paulo Freire, Pedagogy of Freedom*. Rowman & Littlefield.

Aronowitz, S. (2008). *Against Schooling: For an Education That Matters*. Paradigm Publishers.
Aronowitz, S. (2009). Foreword. In S. L. Macrine (Ed.), *Critical Pedagogy in Uncertain Times: Hope and Possibilities*. Palgrave Macmillan.
Bibby, T. (2011). *Education—An 'Impossible Profession'? Psychoanalytic Explorations of Learning and Classrooms*. Routledge.
Biesta, G. (2006). *Beyond Learning: Democratic Education for a Human Future*. Routledge.
Britzman, D. (1991). *Practice Makes Practice: A Critical Study of Learning to Teach*. SUNY Press.
Britzman, D. (2015). *A Psychoanalyst in the Classroom*. SUNY Press.
Cho, D. (2009). *Psychopedagogy: Freud, Lacan, and the Psychoanalytic Theory of Education*. Palgrave Macmillan.
Clarke, M., & Kennedy, A. (2024). A Psychosocial Reading of Teacher Agency. *Teachers and Teaching*, 1–16. https://doi.org/10.1080/13540602.2024.2401090
Copjec, J. (2015). *Read My Desire. Lacan Against the Historicists*. Verso.
Coveney, P. (1967). *The Image of Childhood*. Penguin.
Cunningham, H. (2005). *Children and Childhood in Western Society Since 1500*. Routledge.
Felman, S. (1982). Psychoanalysis and Education: Teaching Terminable and Interminable. *Yale French Studies, 63*, 21–44.
Freire, P. (1993). *Pedagogy of the Oppressed*. Penguin.
Freire, P. (2014). *Pedagogy of Hope*. Bloomsbury Academic.
Giroux, H. A. (2010). Rethinking Education as the Practice of Freedom: Paulo Freire and the Promise of Critical Pedagogy. *Policy Futures in Education, 8*(6), 715–721.
Hursh, D. (2018). The Rise of Authoritarian Neoliberalism: How Neoliberalism Threatens Public Education and Democracy. In *Challenges for Public Education* (pp. 145–158). Routledge.
Malabou, C. (2010). *Plasticity at the Dusk of Writing*. Columbia University Press.
Malabou, C. (2012). *Ontology of the Accident: An Essay on Destructive Plasticity* (C. P. T. Shread, Ed.). Polity.
Malabou, C. (2023). *Stop Thief! Anarchism and Philosophy*. Polity.
Pagès, A. (2025). Teaching as an act: Lacan and philosophy of education. *Journal of Philosophy of Education, qhaf021*.Chicago
Rancière, J. (1991). *The Ignorant Schoolmaster: Five Lessons in Intellectual Emancipation*. Stanford University Press.
Reshe, J. (2017). The Changing Child. *Knowledge Cultures, 5*(2), 163–177.
Reshe, J. (2023). *Negative Psychoanalysis for the Living Dead. Philosophical Pessimism and the Death Drive*. Palgrave Macmillan.

Robertson, S. L., & Nestore, M. (2021). Education Cleavages, or Market Society and the Rise of Authoritarian Populism? *Globalisation, Societies and Education, 20*(2), 110–123.

Rose, J. (1985). Introduction II. In J. Mitchell & J. Rose (Eds.), *Feminine Sexuality: Jacques Lacan and the École Freudienne* (pp. 27–57). W.W. Norton & Co..

Rossatto, C. A. (2002). Critical Pedagogy Applied Praxis: A Freirean Interdisciplinary Project and Grassroot Social Movement. *Counterpoints, 209*, 157–171.

Salajan, F. D., & Jules, T. D. (2024). The Global Resurgence of Authoritarianism and Its Existential Threats to Education: Implications for Scholarship in Comparative and International Education. *Comparative Education Review, 68*(3), 319–344.

Watts, J. (Ed.). (1977). *The Countesthorpe Experience*. Allen and Unwin.

Webster, J. (2022). *Disorganization and Sex*. Divided.

Zapffe, P. W. (1933). The Last Messiah. 'Den sidste Messias'. *Janus, 9*, 645–665.

CHAPTER 6

The Jouissance of Teaching

Abstract Beginning with an account of the horrors of modern teaching, this final chapter offers the possibility of remaining as a classroom teacher that finds enjoyment beyond the signifier of lack and sadomasochism raised in prior chapters. A thorough examination of Lacan's concept of jouissance is given that leads into alternative modes of enjoyment. One mode is the tragic, drawing on Nietzche, Malabou and others, posing the subject of the teacher as one who has accepted the end of education. This figure is further explored through the example of Bartleby and beyond. The chapter moves from tragedy to alienation via the work of Brecht and Lacan's founding of a new psychoanalytic school, giving further examples of Lacan's own modes of pedagogy. The finals sections of the chapter raise the enjoyment of speech as lalangue or 'blahblahblah', found in Joyce and the hysterical subject.

Keywords Enjoyment • jouissance • Lack • Death drive • Tragedy • Lalangue • Hysteria • Teacher • Teaching • Classroom • Sadomasochism • Bartleby • Theatre • Repetition • Alienation • Pedagogy • Signifier • Deconstruction

I explain nothing.
—(Jacques Lacan, Seminar XVI, p. 139)

© The Author(s), under exclusive license to Springer Nature Switzerland AG 2025

N. Stock, N. Peim, *The Lacanian Teacher*, The Palgrave Lacan Series, https://doi.org/10.1007/978-3-031-93018-8_6

Classroom Jouissance

Are teachers enjoying themselves? National education has been a concern for politicians for the past century, though particularly in the UK there have been more overt interventions in the past few decades into the education system that many teachers (perhaps falsely) believe pose a threat to its integrity. Absurd demands for 'our schools' to take on all sorts of social ills proliferate from all quarters. Always at the centre of public debate, the demand is repeatedly made that teachers must remain politically neutral (DfE, 2022) in an institution that is fundamentally political in its history and structure (Donald, 1992; Hunter, 1994; Peim, 2022). Many have also noted an authoritarian shift in the profession (Reay, 2022; Clarke, 2023), both in classroom practice and in government policy. Inspection remains a looming predatory figure, commonly cited as one of the largest pressures for teaching staff and management, even a source of anxiety (Poole, 2023). Poor funding, endless planning, preparation, marking, data gathering, and general administrative workloads, alongside the continued rise in teacher observation, surveillance and performance management (Clarke & Phelan, 2017), pushed the sector (and its university cousins) into a wave of national (and international) strikes (Flores, 2023) that were demonstrably ineffective in shifting political opinions with the media regularly portrayed teachers as lazy, entitled and greedy. Numerous schools report a misogynistic turn in male student behaviour, with the 'manosphere' and 'incel community' becoming an apparent threat to teachers (Stahl et al., 2022). Huge numbers are leaving the profession (Clarke & Phelan, 2017; Ellis, 2024), and recruitment targets regularly fall short of the required numbers—surely signs that there is little to enjoy in being a teacher.

But then again, psychoanalysis makes us look at what is pleasurable or enjoyable slightly differently. Might there be enjoyment here in the teachers' complaints? Lacan recognised that acts of masochism are a 'practice of jouissance' (XVI, p. 95): the daily suffering of teachers in the name of education might conceivably be an unconscious form of enjoyment. We have also seen in the fantasies of 'by any means necessary', a certain strain of classroom sadism might exist in the teachers who find enjoyment in berating or belittling their students for educational 'goods', now armed with even greater performative and accountability measures for their cause. So too, as we have claimed in the previous two chapters, might the very act of teaching in its non-lacking fantasy of the pedagogical relationship be an act of enjoyment by occupying the fraudulent position of the knowing subject. What we will start to explore here, in working through enjoyment, is whether other forms might be out there for the teacher beyond the signifier of lack and the sadomasochistic.

Though we often use the term interchangeably in this book, and as we started to suggest in an earlier chapter, enjoyment does not quite encapsulate what Lacan means by *jouissance*. The concept shifts throughout Lacan's teachings, tracked by Jacques-Alain Miller as six different 'paradigms of jouissance' (2019b). Rather than trying to work through the difference in each paradigm or synthesise all six, we will deploy the term more flexibly, ultimately to make it clear that there are different ways of obtaining jouissance. After all, enjoying oneself comes in many different forms, and as such this can be true for the teacher too. Still, there are features to jouissance in its different paradigms that are worth highlighting here. Lacanian analyst and translator of Lacan Bruce Fink claims that:

> The moment in which one seeks therapy can thus be understood as one in which a breakdown occurs in that person's favorite or habitual way of obtaining jouissance. It is a "jouissance crisis". (1999, p. 9)

Jouissance extends beyond the merely pleasurable answering to what is found in meeting the needs of the drives. To use the previous example of anality and its drive: when one needs to defecate, the shitting is pleasurable. Staying on the toilet for too long, long after need has been met, is moving into the realm of pleasure. But jouissance goes a step further: it must extend beyond the meeting of needs *and* desires. *Jouir*, a climactic event, one that is both pleasurable and painful, lacking use, quickly dissipated. Our experience of jouissance is also coupled with the law (XX, p. 3), allocated by it, even. For Lacan there is no enjoyment without the law (meant in its most abstract sense, as in how we might refer to the 'law of nature' or 'the law of the jungle' and so on). It is here we should recall Barthes's words: 'the teacher escapes neither the theatre of speech nor the Law played out on its stage' (1977a, p. 192). On the stage of the classroom, the teacher is beholden to the stage's own Symbolic law that the teacher cannot but speak aloud. The classroom is a space that will offer its own form of (law-related) jouissance to the subjects that sit within it.

We might look again to Freud's famous description of his grandson's 'Fort Da' game here in *Beyond the Pleasure Principle* (SE XVIII) to help further grasp how jouissance is staged. In parallel with his treatment of ex-soldiers, Freud observed his grandson exhibiting behaviours that emphasised a pursuit of suffering within a repetitious structure. He witnessed the young boy throwing a wooden reel with a string into his curtained cot, exclaiming 'fort' [gone] as it disappeared, only to pull it back out again and shout 'a joyful da [there]' (p. 15). The game of 'disappearance and return' (p. 15) was repeated by the boy, and it seemed that he found the second act of the return the more joyful of the two. Freud noticed that the boy was consumed by the *compulsion to repeat* the game, and the very logic of the game was predicated on repetition—something must be lost to derive the pleasure of its return. One must lose it again to gain it again; but it turns out there was more fort than da, an enjoyable withholding of the desired object in the excitation of the anxiety of its loss under controlled conditions. Freud ventured that the boy was repeating an unconscious trauma: his 'mother's departure' (p. 15) in the form of the reel so to master the traumatic event. Lacan pushes further: 'This game … manifests in its radical traits the determination that the human animal receives from the symbolic order' (E, pp. 34–35)—that is, a call for us to enjoy (Copjec, 2015, p. 3), but an enjoyment that is always coupled with its own form of suffering. The game is staged not to generate and then satisfy desire but to replay the condition of desiring, to *stage* desire. The game, in its compulsive nature, affords being in that state of desiring that is both pleasure and pain: or a kind of neither, a state of lack that Lacan finds in language and in every subject: 'language is what hollows being into desire' (Eagleton, 1986, p. 97).

The staging of repetition becomes central to jouissance here; Miller even goes so far as to say 'repetition is repetition of jouissance' (2019b, p. 44). We need not dwell on it, but the acts of the teacher are repetitious at every level, both temporally and in act. Every new academic year the reset button is pushed: a new cohort arrives, there's a new start, actually a restart, on the syllabus, the assessments are staged again on the calendar, the weekly meetings repeat. Enunciations are reiterated in the weekly meetings and in general staffroom discourse. The timetable ensures that the weekly order is repeated through the year. A common mantra for more experienced teachers is that the latest pedagogic fad or teaching tool is 'the same shit in different boxes'. Still, in spite of the complaints of repetition, teachers often remain resistant to the radically new. They might say no to introducing new texts or concepts beyond what they have done before, or are resistant to moving classrooms, changing buildings. Perhaps there is some strange enjoyment in the humdrum cycle of the school. The possibility of slipping into a rhythm that both gives cause for enjoyable complaint and yields annual sufferings might be a masochistic jouissance. We could go further and ask: what might educators be repressing that they repeat in the classroom? What fantasy or real event in their personal history are they reenacting in the educational space of, say, the classroom? Once again, jouissance is certainly already lurking around.

Approaching jouissance another way, we might follow Joan Copjec's (2015) example of the modernist architect Le Corbusier. In his 1923 tract *Towards a New Architecture* Corbusier proposed that utility should be placed at the front and centre of architecture as opposed to decoration, adornment and excess. The educational Symbolic order as it stands in the contemporary moment embodies similar ideas, in that the utilitarian, instrumentalised or performative aspects of education have been placed at the forefront of modern schooling (Clarke & Phelan, 2017)—something clearly enjoyed by politicians, bureaucrats, and educational resource companies that thrive off this ever-expanding capitalist agenda. Le Corbusier's important addendum to his architectural maxim, however, was that things of utility might also yield pleasure. One need only look at the Villa Savoye or the Marseille Housing Unit designed by Corbusier to see how this could be so: simplicity and functionality of the form makes them pleasurable. Some will, I imagine, argue similar points about pedagogy. That in its simplest, most didactic and instrumentalist form, there is pleasure to be found. Those of us who enjoy attending classic lectures with a clear understanding that we are learning to pass an exam would embody this space, such as in the 2006 film *The Ron Clark Story* cited a few times in this book. The film regularly repeats the mantras that learning is 'fun' and that 'maximising test scores' is paramount—a deliberate tying of jouissance to the monotonous business of passing exams, manifest in the final scene where the students receive the highest test scores in the state.

Lacan, however, inverts Le Corbusier's maxim that utility can have pleasure as is manifest in the 'International' architecture of the modernist movement, noting in turn that pleasure can have utility. It is here we find something many teachers regularly profess and perhaps contend is where their enjoyment lies: that students will find some pleasure in their learning, even if it is for the tedious utilitarian function of the neoliberal schooling age, and that the teacher will enjoy seeing the student 'reach their potential' or 'fall in love with a text' despite the demands of classroom law. But jouissance would stretch much further than this slightly glib claim that teachers should simply aim to bring more pleasure into their classrooms to enable more educational utility. Indeed, the teachers that expound these 'pleasure plus utility' pedagogies are perhaps even more troubling than the former simply utilitarian ones, again seen in *Ron Clark* as the eponymous hero downs carton after carton of chocolate milk whilst teaching his students grammar in the promise that he might 'puke' for their pleasure if they just listen to some teaching. Jouissance cannot be tethered to learning like this for it is, ultimately 'what serves no purpose' (XX, p. 3). This is why it is so difficult to think about in the Symbolic order of education that priorities the utility of knowledge, instrumentality or progress. Even in the commonly cited myth of an education without utility, where learning is for learning's sake, the very notion of the 'sake' is a purpose in itself. This might yield pleasure, but not enjoyment. Such formulations touch on the very Lacanian split between the desire to impose an order like curriculum specifications, key stages, litter-free schools, and so on, and the activation at the same time of the innumerable strands of desire that in turn animate jouissance. Perhaps, however, if we saw Ron Clark puking in a classroom for the explosion alone, an absurdist beyond of classroom law, we might be into the realms of new modes of jouissance (Clark of course keeps all the milk down).

What threads entangle the moment of jouissance and the structure of pedagogy? For example, those who claim to make lessons 'fun' and 'exciting', usually through a game or distracting activity, evidence a need to turn pleasure into utility and thus fall back into the fantasy of educational redemption, or into neoliberal fantasies of future career success, a form of jouissance that arises when one believes something has been purposefully completed. We find this even in the pleasure felt when a school receives a 'Good' or above rating from Ofsted or a similar inspectorate. But the more powerful Lacanian insight to the notion that pleasure can have utility, however, is not that we can deploy pleasure for utilitarian ends, but that we do not and cannot know what pleasure it is that we seek. For the subject, whether that be teacher, student, or anyone else, 'being subject to a principle beyond pleasure, is not driven to seek his own good' (Copjec, 2015, p. 87). We would argue that this paradox pertains to the teacher more so than many other positions in society. For the teacher, even the most cynical one, is the subject who, when pressed on who they are and what they do, tends to claim to seek good through the act of education. The fantasies so common in the educational Imaginary outlined in Chap. 3, 'making a difference', 'enriching lives', or 'having a meaningful role in society', are problematised by jouissance: it remains always-already coloured by its masochism, its self-destruction. As such the teacher cannot seek good for all, as they cannot know 'the good' that exists beyond their pleasure. Even the very notion of 'good', in psychoanalytic terms, can be inflected with much darker and more taboo desires.

Jouissance is a problem for articulation, a problem in the order of education, something that remains generally unspoken, for there is often shame in what we enjoy, especially as it often lies outside of the big Other's dictates of sanctioned zones of enjoyment. As such 'People repress said jouissance because it is not fitting' (XX, p. 61) or 'proper' (as Fink says in the fn.p. 61). We might think of the teacher who berates the student, visibly finding enjoyment in the negative exchange. Any teacher who has taught on a corridor on a summer's day with all the classroom doors open knows this moment, when an explosion of vitriol assaults a student who didn't 'listen' to what the teacher believed they were saying. In the voice lies the traces of jouissance. The listening to the teacher was only ever a precursor to the enjoyment found in violence towards the student who didn't listen. But the teacher could never admit it. Catch that teacher later on in the day: 'It was awful, but I had to do it. She's not been listening to me all year, and with her exams around the corner it's essential that she listens to me. This was the only way', says the teacher, parroting the stance of the big Other. Ultimately, the jouissance speaks even if the subject does not: 'jouissance would do better to hush up' (XX, p. 61). But it does not hush up, of course, as the pedagogy will keep on going. 'I know I shouldn't have gone on that tangent in the lesson, but it's really important that students know these things!' some teachers say becoming in that moment a subject who knows, even if that knowledge is not curricular, but perhaps is more powerfully about 'life'. In such instances we may find that pedagogy functions as one of many 'apparatuses of jouissance' (XX, p. 55).

From the position of the subject—the teacher, say—they also believe that the Other is experiencing jouissance in a manner that they desire. If we are not experiencing enough ourselves, we presume that the Other is stealing jouissance—that they are experiencing something that we cannot, and thus we must refind our own in the rejection, oppression, or demonisation of that Other. As in Said's (2003) landmark theory of Orientalism, the common examples of fetishization of race or class or sexuality are clear embodiments of this structure, though it is interesting in a classroom to consider how the teacher might experience anger or jealousy for the enjoyment of the Other. Commonly we see the contempt the teacher feels for the student who doesn't want to learn, a contempt that extends to the unseen image of a perceived inferior culture or mode of being. Contemptuous expressions like 'Do you want to work in McDonalds when you leave school?' are commonplace, only aggravated further by the reluctant learner's indifference towards the apparatus of education and enjoyment of 'so much else'. Lacan's peer Solange Faladé (1996) examined, in a similar manner, how race functions in this mode of enjoyment. As such, it is no surprise that similar logics will pertain in the classroom. This is especially the case in the classroom space that makes strong claims to being a place of equality, fairness, non-judgement and anti-racism. As always with the perspective, it is precisely in this claim that we are likely to find the most oppressive and divisive behaviours. As Richards notes in his presentation of Lacan and Faladé, 'any attempt to force a homogeneous cultural context or environment, preventing jouissance for anybody, and any attempt to oblige such a homogeneous cultural context is racist, a stifling violence' (2023, p. 442). The classroom in its most authoritarian Imaginary is easy to insert into Richard's argument here, where the necessity to homogenise students as subjects of pedagogy—as *learners*, will always be an act of stifling violence and a theft of jouissance.

We, therefore, do not think there is a jouissance crisis in education, no 'breakdown ... in [teachers'] favorite or habitual way of obtaining jouissance' (Fink, 1999, p. 9). Teachers find all manner of ways of enjoyment through educational means. Indeed, numerous studies of would-be teachers find similar things repeatedly, even in spite of the supposedly shifting educational landscape. Teachers almost always report a desire for passion, fun, and enjoyment in their pursuit of teaching as a career, and even if it is not always readily found, there is a clear *possibility* of it being uncovered (Lortie, 1975; Britzman, 1991; Schutz et al., 2001; Bergmark et al., 2018; Gorard et al., 2023). What our chapter on fantasies proffered was that this enjoyment is felt through the embodiment of the fantasies that encircle the teacher as a subject. Only, we portend, these fantasies act as powerful vehicles for modes of enjoyment that are commonly infused with the non-lacking, the sadistic, and the masochistic. So too do they uphold an educational Imaginary that does (at least Symbolic) violence to staff, students and the society it supposedly redeems. How is one to teach and find enjoyment then, if not submitting oneself to authoritarian desire, sadomasochism, Symbolic violence, or fraudulent possession of the signifier of lack? The answer cannot be to simply close the schools and universities, stop education, an end to education, can it? Not for us, because as we have implied throughout the book, the space and relationships of education are fascinating places where there is much of intrigue happening. The trouble comes in trying to work through what they are without slipping into the tropes of liberatory pedagogy or other educational alternatives. A brief return to Lacan's graph of desire in Seminar XX alerts us to the possibility, he says, of an Other jouissance beyond that of the signifier of lack that is demanded of us in the pedagogised space of our subjectivity. In the graph of sexuation, this Other jouissance, one that is not revolving around the function of the signifier of lack but finds its enjoyment somewhere unknowable. We hope to find the same for the teacher.

Towards Tragedy

In *Seminar VII*, Lacan gives his famous maxim regarding the ethics of psychoanalysis, that 'the only thing of which one can be guilty is of having given ground relative to one's desire' (VII, p. 392). There are different ways of reading this maxim, though. We see it as an important call to reject the desire of the big Other and seek one's own desire, a task that will entail freeing oneself from the demands of the law, the signifier of the master (and indeed the university, the school, education…). Lacan's great example is Sophocles's *Antigone,* where the eponymous young woman defies King Creon's orders by burying her brother Polyneices, an act that leads to her tragic death. She appears to us as 'crossing the barrier of the city, the law, the barrier of the beautiful, into the zone of horror that jouissance implies' (Miller, 2019b, p. 30). The disobedience of Antigone in her pursuit of her desire thus upholds Lacan's maxim (though there are clearly issues with how she submits to a law of familial obligation instead). Though not always read as a tragedy, Ibsen's *A Doll's House* might stand as another example. Nora Helmer, a woman who initially appears to live a contented life in a seemingly perfect marriage, leaves her husband to pursue what she claims is her freedom. The desire here though really lingers in the madness of the act. She likely leaves her husband to enter into destitution so to free herself from the oppression of patriarchy: more so than Antigone, she crosses a (physical) barrier into the realm of horror. Her desire becomes an act of jouissance, a going beyond the laws that are preached to Nora by her husband at the close of the play. In both of these examples, tragedy becomes entangled with jouissance, a staging of both pain and pleasure without redemption and thus without cause. This is not news to those who are interested in psychoanalysis, with Freud's mapping of the narrative of *Oedipus Rex* and *Hamlet* onto the familial structure and psyche (SE XIV) demonstrating a clear investment in tragedy as fundamental to psychoanalytic thought. Indeed, Lacan went on to note that 'tragedy is in the forefront of our experiences as analysts' (VII, p. 243).

We've argued elsewhere (Peim, 2016; Stock, 2020) that philosophy stands in an interesting and important, non-identical relation to tragedy (and education), and Lacan's interest in *Antigone, Hamlet, Oedipus* and tragedy broadly echoes this in the psychoanalytic sphere. The dimension of the tragic, in terms of what Greek tragedy stages, as it were, in ontological terms, is attuned to and acknowledged in certain modes of modern philosophy, including the Lacanian. But tragedy is also, to a significant degree, what philosophy and western metaphysics has eschewed, as a disturbance to the rationalist project that seeks to determine the nature and limits of things through the application of a mode of thinking that can stabilize the free play of the signifier in ordered and decisive chains of meaning. This process effectively subsumes the ontological force of the category of jouissance as the essential companion to the drive. Put differently by Zupančič, tragedies 'give body to a certain impasse of desire, as well as to a certain way of dealing with this impasse' (2003, p. 174). We might rephrase again by saying that there is something of the Real breaking through the neatness of the Symbolic order in the staging of tragedy.

Nietzsche's *Birth of Tragedy* (1872) traces a significant shift in Greek sensibility from the era of classic Attic tragedy to the moment of Socrates and Euripides, representing these two in a secret collaboration to render its Promethean force amenable to rational thought, control and intelligibility, a difference that has a kind of parallel in Lacan's schema set against the pretensions of instrumental rationality. We could see this as the aim of bringing tragedy into the classroom as a curricula object. In choosing to teach *Oedipus at Colonus* for the means of English or classics education, it is ordered neatly in the Symbolic process of progress and improvement: tragedy is made 'good for you', vital to the improvement of the human animal.

In *The Birth of Tragedy* Nietzsche suggests tragedy (beyond a certain form of dramatic practice) entails a way of thinking and being-in-the-world, an attunement to being that eschews any overriding principle of reason, any recourse to ready-to-hand rationality, perhaps any falling into the desire of the big Other. Tragedy in this sense seems to be attuned to the Lacanian perspective that refuses to hold out false promises of redemption, salvation or any final therapeutic settlement for the barred subject (Webster, 2022). The Lacanian mode of thinking, with its ontological division into the Imaginary, Symbolic and Real, and with its insistence on the implacability of the unconscious, like tragedy in the Nietzschean sense, engenders and demands 'negative capability', constantly reiterating the relation between the realms of meaning, action and death. Tragedy stages the relations between presence and absence, between past and present as disturbed by trauma, problematizing rationalist models of knowledge and meaning. In tragedy reason is always beset by some attendant madness, the irrationality of the barred subject beset by the unconscious and, in the register of desire, entrammelled in the play of the signifier. What's more, both tragedy and the Lacanian perspective acknowledge that the very order of things is predicated on fundamental trauma, an always disturbing possibility that has already happened. As Zupančič notes, tragedy stages the 'price the subject has to pay to get access to … the Real' that which 'constitutes the very kernel of the subject's being, the kernel that is simultaneously created and extirpated by the advent of the signifying order' (2003, p. 174). As such, both tragedy and Lacan similarly warn against complacent confidence in the order of things, in one's own knowledge and in aspirations to 'mastery'.

As may be obvious, in tragedy death is staged: mourning, loss and grief are the order of the day and provide a constant palpable backdrop to everyday commerce. Tragedy, thus equipped with 'the ontology of the accident' (Malabou, 2012) warns against overinvestment in the blandishments of lucid rationality that lure us into complacent faith in the order of things. That way hubris lies. Tragedy—not theatre, nor misfortune, but the particular, peculiar quality of Attic tragedy—constitutes an 'orientation to meaning' and an orientation to being at odds with the instrumental rationalist tendencies, ensconced in institutional practices and curricula that have dominated educational thinking and practice with its means-ends logic (Heidegger, 1977). Tragedy properly disdains any overarching ethic of redemption driven by such rationalist hubris. As Catherine Malabou might put it, 'destructive plasticity' (2010, 2012), as an inescapable dimension of being, must recognize that all flourishings and becomings are subject to catastrophic reversal or to termination. If this seems obvious, Malabou (drawing significantly on both Hegel and Heidegger) indicates how the dominant metaphysics of our era has consistently foreclosed the destructive element in plasticity as Julie Reshe has insisted (Malabou, 2010; Reshe, 2023).

While Plato sought to banish the tragic poets from the ideal state, Aristotle sought to redefine tragedy as collective therapy, still it is clear from frequent references that tragedy reverberates with Lacanian ontology. Nietzsche similarly sets the Dionysian, one of his twin poles of tragedy, essential other to the Apollonian, against what he refers to as the 'satisfaction and serenity of the theoretical man' (Nietzsche, 1872, p. 4). Tragedy belongs to the projected world of the symbolic in its encounter with the formless and terrifying real, problematizing the strictures of instrumental rationality that dominate modernity with its 'technological enframing' where the essence of technology—itself a kind of positive reduction of truth—is negated in the pursuit of resource in an equation of being with productivity and investment value.

Plato's desire to expel the tragic poets from the Republic appears as an attempt to banish the aporias of tragedy as what threatens clarity of thought. Tragedy can only claim a space in the republic's vision of the polis if it can demonstrate that, like philosophy, it can 'calm down' and be subjected to Aristotle's abstracted poetics, philosophy's therapeutic triumph over tragedy. Shouldn't we be suspicious of this separation of philosophy from tragedy and of the attempt to render tragedy—a 'hot' medium—into the cool rationality of one modality of philosophy. Tragedy frequently problematizes the cool and rational search for truth, putting the aporetic, the agonistic into play as essential, driving components. Tragedy acknowledges that techniques of sophistry are mobilized in discourse, staging arguments and counter arguments that are always strongly positioned and rooted in specific metaphysics.

When tragedy arises as a question for philosophy in modernity with Nietzsche and with Heidegger, but also emphatically with Freud and Lacan, the register of tragedy returns to philosophy. The question of a relation to tragedy—or at least to the problematizations that tragedy brings with it—becomes 'fundamental' to the project of philosophy. In the legacy of Aristotle, Hegel and Rousseau, philosophy seeks to explain and ultimately to rationalize and domesticate the meaning of tragic experience. Tragedy is conceived of as a cleansing agent, a kind of emotional balm, offering a therapeutic engagement with the dubious and problematic that will ultimately give rise to engagement with the clear realm of rational thought proper.

Tragedy is Lacanian in staging the interplay between Imaginary, Symbolic and Real, the indeterminate, overlaid spaces of Lacanian ontology. Tragedy foregrounds the role of the Symbolic in its disturbing difference from the Real. Tragedy is founded in this difference and can be thought of as the very medium of radical difference and aporia. In tragedy, action is predicated on undecidability and the madness of decision. Tragedy renders action both undecidable and 'mad' subverting the cool calculations of reason. The drive is foregrounded while any reason in action is permeated with desire born of the difference between the symbolic and the real, foregrounding the unreason of decision and the tragedy of responsibility in staging the condition of undecidability that attends action. The provenance of the aporetic qualifies the overweening, ego-bound claims of reason and puts it in its limited place. As such, tragedy expresses an essential condition of collective life (Vernant & Vidal-Naquet, 1990). It problematizes any simple, ontotheological relation to our prized rationality whether it be individual or collective hence its frequent representation of madness as being the essential companion of reason. The social subject is the subject, at the same time, of jouissance, driven by the self-annihilating desire fuelled by Symbolic commitments, as with Oedipus, Clytemnestra, Antigone or Orestes. What tragedy stages as such is a working through of the '"fear of castration"... the fear of losing that which constitutes a signifying support for the lack involved in the experience of the desire as such' (Zupančič, 2003, p. 178). In accepting oneself as lacking, not possessing any signifier of lack, we might see the seeds of unsettling jouissance in the educational Symbolic order where the relentless demand for the jouissance of non-lack occurs.

We are aware that there is some slippage above between the ethics of desire and the affect of jouissance. While desire and jouissance are not the same, engaging with Lacan's ethics of psychoanalysis regarding desire opens up the possibility of new forms of jouissance. As Miller alerts us to in *Paradigms of Jouissance*, 'Jouissance in one respect is nothing other than desire, which is at the same time dead desire' (2019b, p. 25). In the pursuit of what is desired, what is 'killed' along the way offers jouissance. In the classroom it entails a rejection (or murder) of the law of the master signifier education. In the ceaseless search for new forms of desire, we might find ourselves somewhere different where new wellsprings of jouissance are opened to us as teachers. As we have made clear throughout this book, the classroom makes this a particularly challenging task: it is a space wherein the very Symbolic structure works to foreclose desires, to repress new wishes, and to repeat archaic fantasies. When we walk into the classroom, we find ourselves saying the things we thought we would never say as teachers. We become teachers, inhabiting that subject position in its relation to the function of the signifier of lack, and continue to enact the educational mission laid out for us by the big Other. To work with this impasse, we might say that if the classroom indeed takes the form of a stage as we have repeatedly asserted, then why not make the performance accord with 'the spirit of tragedy'? In this move, as a radical rejection of and striving beyond the law of education, we project an acceptance of the castration of the teacher, and indeed new possibilities of different forms of jouissance that go beyond the law. As Cioran says, there is 'Nothing more alien to tragedy than the notion of redemption, of salvation, of immortality' (2018, p. 87). Theo-educational laws, the will to save, redeem, complete the subject, are rejected in the mode of tragedy. What is left for the teacher that rejects them?

The Figure of Death

Beyond the narrative of tragedy, Žižek offers a compelling depiction of the Lacanian ethical imperative through the example of Melville's *Bartleby*. The story is narrated by the lawyer who employs Bartleby, who confesses to being intrigued and concerned by his enigmatic conduct. In an important sense, it seems, Bartleby puzzles him in a non-trivial way, disturbing his sense of the order of things in his inexplicable attitude and demeanour. Eventually Bartleby gets left behind as the lawyer moves office, at a loss to deal with Bartleby, abandoning his former scrivener to his fate, an apparent torpor without end that leads to death, leaving the lawyer dwelling darkly on human fate.

Bartleby exerts a fascination for theorists who sense something important is going on in the narrative of faint refusal. For us, the figure Bartleby and the narrative of *Bartleby the Scrivener*, exemplify importantly discomfiting aspects of the pedagogical scene, and, metonymically, of the educational enterprise, disturbing the educational logic that so frequently presents itself as self-explanatory, as common-sensical, as so obvious and proper as to be self-evident, despite the constant injunctions that appear to be required to keep it going—in assemblies, in prospectuses, and in all the casual or sustained daily harangues of teachers and teaching to get things done, to avoid wasting time, to be productive, to make something of your time and of yourself. Bartleby stands out, however, as the scrivener who, while initially performing the role, appears to not want to work as a scrivener, to do no scrivening. Beyond that, Bartleby sinks into a condition of enigmatic reverie (or is it blankness?), staring aimlessly at a wall, unreachable, apparently beyond communication except to reiterate his negative desire, to the point where he ceases to be a scrivener and sinks into a state of inertia.

Bartleby has been read in a number of ways, most commonly perhaps as a commentary on the new world order represented by Wall Street in the story, Bartleby's refusal being read a form of appropriate passive resistance. But Bartleby doesn't refuse in the name of some other, non-instrumental, non-bureaucratic more positive, creative mode of being: the meaning of his 'passive resistance' remains enigmatic and leads only to disconnection and death. Bartleby's condition has been variously pathologized—as depression, anorexia, agoraphobia—to make sense of the story's trajectory and significance. It has been read as an indictment of economic instrumentalism, being explicitly labelled as *A Story of Wall Street*. Towards the very end, it is revealed that there has been a rumour concerning Bartleby alleging that he had worked at the 'Dead Letter Office' that seems to give the tale a much more ontological inflection.

Žižek recognises the complexity of this tale, too, finding the trace of Lacan's ethical imperative:

> His "I would prefer not to" is to be taken literally: it says "I would prefer not to," not "I don't prefer (or care) to" ... In his refusal of the Master's order, Bartleby does not negate the predicate; rather, he affirms a non-predicate: he does not say that *he doesn't want to do it;* he says that he *prefers (wants) not to do it*. This is how we pass from the politics of "resistance" or "protestation," which parasitizes upon what it negates, to a politics which opens up a new space outside the hegemonic position and its negation. We can imagine the varieties of such a gesture in today's public space: not only the obvious "There are great chances of a new career here! Join us!"—"I would prefer not to"; but also "Discover the depths of your true self, find inner peace!"—"I would prefer not to"; or "Are you aware how our environment is endangered? Do something for ecology!"—"I would prefer not to"; or "What about all the racial and sexual injustices that we witness all around us? Isn't it time to do more?"—"I would prefer not to." This is the gesture of subtraction at its purest, the reduction of all qualitative differences to a purely formal minimal difference. (Žižek, 2009, pp. 381–2)

In this reading, it would be tempting to imagine this Bartleby-like subject in the educational Symbolic as one that simply slacks off, does nothing, rejects what they are impelled to do. Certainly, there is 'some enjoyment from secretly slacking off and rebelling against the Other's desire' (Swales, 2023, p. 24), a form of jouissance that many are doubtless already pursuing at times. It is a great joy to give out 'the laptops' to a class at the end of the day with a fairly idle task, one that neither you nor the students care is completed. You sit and stare at the classroom, enjoying the appearance of work from the students in parallel with the lack of productivity from anyone in the room. However, as Swales (p. 24) points out, in the Symbolic order of work (like that of the office or indeed the school), the superego will come to prey on you eventually. The enjoyment quickly becomes guilt or malaise, a symptom that is harder to manage, so we must note that Bartleby is not simply the figure of the slacker. It is not that he can't be bothered, but that he would prefer not to. Bartleby manages to exploit a 'rupture in the symbolic chain' (Miller, 2019b, p. 18), a hole that he can dwell in that brings forth jouissance.

We might reread Bartleby as exemplifying, in extreme form, the Lacanian death drive (or drive): as in the end and through much of the tale's duration Bartleby appears as 'a shell which remains after it is deprived of its substance' (Reshe, 2023, p. 26) or as Julie Reshe translates it the barred subject, $. This is the subject 'who …' in Žižekian terms drawn from Lacan 'continues to live after it is deprived of its substance' (p. 26). The ontological dimension is perhaps obvious here, if obviously pessimistic. Lacan asserts that in the human 'there's already a crack, a perturbation of the regulation of life. That's the importance of the notion introduced by Freud of the death instinct' (quoted in Reshe, 2023, p. 36) a notion that acknowledges that in the break between symbolic and real there comes into play another kind of logic of life. This other logic of life opens the difference between the subject as such and the subject as identified in and through the Symbolic order. This is the disparity introduced by language, the difference that separates living substance and the domain of meaning.

Bartleby is upbraided by the lawyer in terms of negating 'common usage', a last resort justification for the demand the lawyer wants to make on Bartleby to be more and other than what his persistent and persistently polite refusal ('I would prefer not to') entails. But Bartleby remains faithful to 'the basic zero-level form of subjectivity' as Julie Reshe has it, that is 'a pure subject of a death drive' (2023, p. 35). But this is no extreme case driven to its limit. Borrowing Malabou's terminology, Reshe affirms that 'the subject as such is already a result of destructive plasticity' and is, like Bartleby, 'a living figure of death' (p. 36). Bartleby represents the stripped-down subject who automaton-like refuses the blandishments of the

Symbolic order, who in some trance-like condition, sees beyond the play of meaning to the brick wall of unmeaning that is its always possible other.

So Bartleby appears as the instantiation of impotentiality, the opposite pole of the productive world of 'common usage' that goes about its pointless business with the air of purpose, disavowing 'the vanity of human wishes' and ultimate 'solar death' through the attachment to the worldly business of everyday life. As Derrida notes, giving us more to think about with Bartleby beyond mere idleness, especially in the role played by this figure in the relationship between analyst and analysand, or between teacher and student:

> Bartleby is a figure of death, to be sure, but they also know how, without saying anything, he makes others speak, above all the narrator, who happens to be a responsible man of the law and a tireless analyst. In truth incurable. Bartleby makes the analyst speak as narrator and man of the law. Bartleby is also the secret of literature. There where perhaps it makes psychoanalysis talk–or sing. (Derrida, 1998, p. 24)

On this appropriately inscrutable reading, Bartleby—enigmatic, indefinable, beyond the touch of utility—is the occasion for the animation of the signifier in the Other. Literature, like Bartleby is useless, and (again like Bartleby) resists all efforts to enclose it within a Symbolic order that will quell its 'secret'.

The lesson of Bartleby is therefore not to do nothing, but rather to reject the demands of the master, refuse the desire of the Other, whilst while being situated in whatever Symbolic order into which you are thrown. Bartleby's refusal, an inherently hysterical act (Webster, 2015, p. 3), a rejection of the symbolic, knots together some of the threads we have explored in this book. Bartleby, then, touches on the 'traumatic heart' of the subject of the death drive and enacts something of its 'disintegrative traumatic core' (Reshe, 2023, p. 37) and a core that makes us speak up. We cannot but 'talk-or sing' (Derrida, 1998, p. 24) when it arises. One upshot of the staging of this figure is to render problematic to the point of impossible the ethical demeanour of the lawyer, who, living within the bounds of 'common usage', is thrown out of joint by the figure of Bartleby, and who in turn is thrown into a morbid state of melancholy concerning 'humanity' ('Ah humanity!'). The figure of Bartleby presents an equally traumatic blow to the ethical pretensions of resistance to the order of things (or 'common usage' as the lawyer has it). Bartleby's refusal is grounded in no apparent principle and leads to no apparent benefit; it simply seems to spring from a death drive inertia that has no telos and that finally gives up on its last vestiges of jouissance ('ginger nuts'). Bartleby's final days are spent in 'the Tombs' indicating that he is—Reshe-like—already dead before death occurs.

On this reading of Melville's tale, there is no prescription for conduct, attitude or orientation. Whatever sense we make of Bartleby, the figure of Bartleby remains in some ineradicable dimension, enigmatic, unknowable and indefinable. The lawyer's incomprehension is the dramatized form of the incomprehension that is always experienced in the face of the other. The impossibility of the relation between subjects is exemplified in stark and troubling form, but it corresponds powerfully with the task and the position of the teacher who is always faced with the other that must be incomprehensible, enigmatic, ultimately unreachable to some degree. What's more, the positive teaching relation, it seems, must be predicated on a shared assumption of the propriety of 'common usage' a propriety that cannot be universally shared and that begins to look like a version of mere surface politeness. If we were, ironically, of course, to take a 'lesson' from Bartleby, it would be to consider the enjoyment or jouissance that might be possible with some accommodation with 'common usage' that doesn't share its inflated pretensions to meaning or necessity.

Lacanian Schools

We have attempted to stress throughout an awareness of the certain impossible but ineradicable features of the Symbolic order of education: its addiction to an ethic of improvement and even of salvation, its implicit commitment to never-ending-progress, its desire to subjectivate students to become saviours not only of themselves but of the future, even ultimately to redeem the world. We recognize this Symbolic order cannot be dismissed from the classroom, just as Bartleby could not dismiss the law of the office. The being of the teacher is predicated on the classroom's enclosure within this fantasmatic space. For the teacher, though, we want to suggest that the possibility of finding enjoyment within it might be a worthy and sufficient project. As we mentioned multiple times in the first chapter, teaching is an 'erotical experience' (Felman, 1982, p. 35), a mode of jouissance. There is just 'something' about it that is hard to find elsewhere. Before Felman, the semiotician Roland Barthes said of the classroom, that it 'is *only* the space of the circulation of subtle desires, mobile desires; it is within the artifice of a sociality whose consistency is miraculously extenuated, according to a phrase of Nietzsche's: "the tangle of amorous relations"' (Barthes, 1977b, p. 171, our emphasis). Drawing on the examples from Lacan's classroom above, and thinking through some of the other aspects of this teaching regarding jouissance and desire, what if this space of subtle desires might be reimagined without the educational impetus that so many of us in the classroom feel compelled to enact? We ask how 'one breaks through the claustrum of ideality' (Britzman, 2015, p. 84).

Lacan was no stranger to these sorts of questions, especially following his expulsion from the International Psychoanalytic Association in 1963. This 'excommunication' was the act of being stripped of the right, or place to teach. As such, Lacan was left with a novel desire—what to teach, how to teach, where to teach? Much of his writing from this period, such as *The Founding Act* or *Seminar XI*, works through this desire. In this process, we find traces of possibilities to explore new modes of enjoyment for the teacher beyond the forms of 'common usage'. Jacques-Alain Miller's work on Lacan's founding of a school in *Turin Theory of the Subject of the School* makes a similar claim. Miller examines Lacan's founding of the *École freudienne de Paris* in 1964, an act that allowed for the position of the teacher within a collective formation to continue, but one that is problematised by the positioning of that figure to the school itself:

> [In 1964, Lacan] advances in the solitude of a subject in relation to a cause to be defended and promoted. He advances presenting himself not as a subject who proposes himself as Ideal but rather as a subject who has a relation to an Ideal, like the others whom he invites to join him in his School. This is not an annulment of the Ideal. There is no annulment of the Ideal in the School. If there were an annulment of the function of the Ideal there would not be a community of the School. There is no zero of the Ideal, but there is this, that Lacan sends each one back to his solitude as a subject, to the relation that each one has with the master signifier of the Ideal beneath which he situates himself. (Miller, 2019a, p. 97)

The 'aim to disassociate' (p. 97) from that very law that governs the school—the ideal, the big Other's imperative to educate, is required in the Lacanian school. Even though Miller here is discussing the more abstracted form of a School of Lacanian psychoanalysis, whose ideal is the desire of

Lacan's to form a new school of psychoanalysis, there is some important transposition to be made. What Miller and Lacan are suggesting is that the law—the educational imperative, the Symbolic order of education, the ideal, cannot be simply erased or elided in some ontological waving of the hand. There remains the necessity of this ideal to engender the very form of the school to take place, and this necessity cannot be abandoned. Like in the opening scene of *Half Nelson* where Mr Dunne teaches his students about the power relations of the classroom, Britzman (1991) gives a telling example of a student teacher who encouraged her students to participate in a discussion about the disciplinary nature of schooling. In doing this, she 'violated a cultural rule by stepping out of her teaching: she attempted to critique the very system, in the eyes of her students, that she represented' (p. 79). This student teacher, in attempting to abolish the Symbolic order of the school, was faced with the big Other's demand that speaks through every corner of the classroom. As such, one cannot abandon or reject the law of the school, but some other form of being within it might be available. Lacan points towards a solitude in the being of the teacher, away from the ideal that forms the school that we have claimed is inescapable, can be recognized. If one wants to teach in a school at all, the ideal must remain, but an 'alienating choice' (p. 98) must be made. It is not to be collectively upheld, as is done in the community of an educational institution as it stands. It is to be situated underneath and dissociated from—remaining in the place of the institution but not in the ego-ideal of the subject within it. Turning again to the pessimism of Emil Cioran, 'A human being possessed by a belief and not eager to pass it on to others is a phenomenon alien to this earth' (2018, p. 5). He too sees the alienation found in this act of moving beyond education's law, breaking free from the 'inferno of saviours' (p. 5).

It is here we might find some resonance again, as in earlier chapters, with the methods of Bertolt Brecht (though Beckett would also be a fruitful example). Brecht perhaps embodies the theoretical insights of Lacan but extends the pedagogy he exemplified in his seminars.[1] Lacan regularly

[1] One might wonder why we opted for Brecht rather than Beckett as the playwright with which we find resonance with Lacanian teaching. Certainly, Beckett's absurdity, his frequent attempts to encapsulate the horror of the Real (in, say, *Waiting for Godot* or *Endgame*), his obsession with the gaze, and his biography (being psychoanalysed himself by Wilfred Bion—an analyst that Lacan respected), would align him with Lacanian thought. Lacan even notes his affinity for Beckett at the start of Seminar XVI when he, alluding to *Endgame*, claims to know 'a bit about garbage cans' (XVI, p. 3). It is also common to see Beckett's famous line

claimed to distance himself from the position of the master in his teaching, even once supposedly proclaiming 'It is up to you to be Lacanians if you wish; I am Freudian.' His reference to himself as a 'clown' (LT), his regular disturbance of the Symbolic space of the teacher, his barbs towards his audience seem to point towards the alienation of the teacher, but one cannot help but feel he continues to pose as an ideal-ego for the students at times—something he may have realised himself in his jokes about being a Messianic or Christ-like figure at the start of *My Teaching* (MT). As we discussed in the previous chapter, Brecht's intentional alienation from the Symbolic law of the stage might provide a similarly fecund model for the teaching, especially when we retain the essential stage-ness of the classroom that we have repeated. His theories of stagecraft and interest in pedagogy (Brecht, 2018, p. 57), particularly in his modes of dialecticization between stage and audience (p. 265), provide interesting models for the being of a teacher (Frimberger, 2022). Brecht in fact goes beyond Lacan in the disturbance of the Symbolic space by refusing the gaze of the audience in its 'continuing search for a reinforcing mirror-image' (Wright, 1989, p. 56). What the audience of a Brechtian play see is the ideal-ego inverted, looking back at the audience and situating them within the performance. Through astonishment, interruption, gesturing, the actor on stage troubles the very act of performance (Benjamin, 1970, pp. 152–152). Each player acts, of course, but acts at acting. Intrusions of strange music, swapping of actors, lines read as if quotation (Jameson, 1998), all contribute to an oddity of the stage, an uncanniness that cannot be ignored in the pursuit of new forms of jouissance in the classroom. Lacan himself was no stranger to this. As Richards makes clear 'Lacan was a surrealist/Dadaist performance artist and spoken word poet' (2024, p. 61). The strangeness of the communication and relentless difficulty of the signifiers, coupled with the meandering detours and ceaseless intertextuality, make for an uncanny performance perhaps better mastered by Brecht.

'Fail again. Fail better' (1983, p. 7) cited in relation to 'radical' education studies (O'Donnell, 2014; Heron & Johnson, 2020). Though some still demand an effort to enfold Beckett into an educational logic, O'Donnell astutely notes that: 'we are inadequate, but we muddle through; the world is a mess, but we should face our situation with courage; education will not change much, but for all that, it is often an enjoyable distraction' (2014, p. 274), with enjoyable being the operative word for us here. Beckett is thus fecund in educational appropriation and requires much more attention, particularly with a psychoanalytic inflection, but Brecht's theories of stagecraft, interest in pedagogy, modes of alienation, and dialecticization are the most relevant to what we discuss here in terms of the performance of the teacher.

Another intriguing thread arises in relation to theatre with Lacan's recognition of himself as a clown, for this opens a possibility beyond both tragic theatre (in its ethical stance) and modernist theatre (in its Brechtian alienation)-comedy and absurdity. Brecht is still a good model here: addressing the bleakest of themes, *Arturo Ui* (1964) comically presents Nazism as gangsters controlling the potato market enhancing the strangeness of that history. As Reshe (2023, p. 83), Zupančič (2008, pp. 28–29) and Critchley (1999) note, 'only comedy is truly tragic' (p. 114). The impotence and jouissance of laughter in the face of being is an expression of hopelessness, another great challenge to the educational project. Lacan stands as the clown of tragic theatre, Lear's fool—'Who is it that can tell me who I am?'—and of comic theatre, Feste once again returning from one of our primal scenes of teaching—'The rain it raineth everyday'. Laughter 'is a disintegrated part of the speech. It is an interruption of speech which acknowledges finitude. It is a convulsive movement that is a testimony to the constitutive rupture of existence' (Reshe, 2023, p. 83). Its convulsiveness and interruption to speech is therefore 'aphonic'. Laughter erupts from the body, usually uncontrollably and without the reliance on the upwards signifying chain. We can laugh in boredom or misery, after all. Of course, it can be pedagogised: making students laugh so that they learn something better is a common teacher trope. This we reject. We emphasise again the necessary estrangement of the tragic mode. One can act on stage as if they are acting, or by parallel, teach on a stage *as if* one were teaching. One can mock one's own performance whilst still playing the part. Even in the "doing" of education, there is possibility of a something else there.

The Letter of the Lesson

As was made clear in the first two chapters, there is much to be gleaned from Lacan's own account of teaching analysts in the space of the classroom, perhaps an example of teaching in an estranged or alienated mode. In *Seminar VIII* on transference, Lacan spends the first half on a lengthy recount and analysis of Plato's *Symposium,* with each session devoted to a different interlocutor and their perspectives on love. It is made clear early on that there is something about love in the way that it is presented in the *Symposium* that interweaves with the phenomenon of transference first discovered by Freud in the Dora analysis. The notion of transference is undoubtedly essential in considering the space of the classroom and the relationship between teacher and student, as comprehensively discussed by Britzman (2015). Continuing the Imaginary analogy of the classroom as a stage we note the metatheatrical moment of Lacan's teaching about transference approximately halfway through the seminar. To quote at length:

> "How did it happen that we are coming to transference so late in the game?" you will ask me.
>
> It is, of course, characteristic of truths to never show themselves completely. In short, truths are solids that are perfidiously opaque. They don't even have, it seems, the property we are able to produce in certain solids, that of transparency—they do not show us their front and back edges at the same time. You have to circumnavigate them, and even do a little conjuring.
>
> As for transference as we are broaching it this year—and you have seen how charmingly I have been able to lead you for a while in making you concern yourselves with love along with me—you must, all the same, have noticed that I approached it from a certain direction or angle, which not only is not the classic angle, but is not even the angle from which I had heretofore approached the topic with you. (VIII, p. 171)

There are important threads to be untangled regarding teaching here: some that point in the direction of new forms of enjoyment; others identify the nature of the classroom but seem trapped by its logic. In this typical, apparently throwaway section from *Seminar VIII*, Lacan refers to the structure of his pedagogy over the course of the preceding sessions. He highlights the concept in hand—here transference, but elsewhere in his career it is the 'sinthome', the gaze, *objet a*, or whatever—but notes that it is only arrived at 'late in the game'. Putting aside the game metaphor of teaching (analogous to our alignment of teaching and theatre), the lateness of the arrival of the concept, is preceded and precipitated by a detour, or as Lacan calls it, being 'able to lead' the listeners 'along with [him]', taking a different or even an obscure 'direction or angle'. Thus far, we might see this as a class pedagogical tactic: the introduction of a concept; a lengthy, seemingly unrelated example; and a punchline or 'big reveal' where the concept is unmasked. But Lacan introduces another dimension: 'truths ... never show themselves completely'. There is no big reveal; only something to be half-understood, malformed from Lacan's own attempt to circumnavigate the opacity of certain truths.

We find this same structure formulated in Lacan's 'Seminar on the Purloined Letter', where Lacan frames 'the letter' as the message that the sender (say, the teacher) wishes to send, the concept they may consciously claim to be sending to the student. But in the unconscious writing of the letter formulating their enunciation, more is written in than the teacher hoped to write or is aware of writing. The unconscious takes on a 'material medium' (E, p. 413) that the sender cannot account for. Lacan goes a step further: the letter is received and read to the letter. Neither sender nor receiver are quite aware of what the intended message was, nor will know what the Other received. Only the way the recipient, the Other, here the student, responds allows the reception of the letter to occur (E, p. 30)—a response that returns the letter to the sender! The letter detours, meandering from the path the sender believed it was to travel.

In the above section on the detour from *Seminar VIII* Lacan finds enjoyment in this detour of the letter. The truth of the concept, the truth of transference in the *Symposium*, say, is traced throughout the letter, but does not become clear or visible in its conclusion. Something else is received by the audience and reflected back at Lacan, just as the words of the teacher are reflected back through the students faces, responses, and work. 'That's not what I said!' cries the exasperated teacher, unable to understand why the students cannot grasp the concept of trochaic tetrameter. But the students heard the teacher: what they heard was a letter consciously unthought by the sender made manifest to the student. Lacan's reframing offers us some alterity, maybe, as in this example, the very detour was as much for the jouissance of the teacher (the 'charmingly' directed teaching) as it was for the learning of the student. Lacan perhaps suggests that what he enjoys in his almost-three decades of teaching, is that the delivery of the letter activates jouissance, not the arrival of the notes made the night before the lesson.

The underlying logic of Lacan's teaching as he describes it in *Seminar VIII* is, of course, that of desire, the metonymic nature of desire that ceaselessly reattaches to a new *objet a*—a process that, Miller claims, becomes an everyday sort of jouissance (2019b, p. 33/41). Jouissance 'inserts itself into the functioning of the signifier' (p. 35), its *function,* not its meaning or signification. In moving constantly from one signifier to the next, signification remains always just out of reach but visible enough to pursue 'an endless series: endless for the reason that every surrogate nevertheless fails to provide the desired satisfaction' (XI, p. 169). Lacan seems to intimate in *Seminar VIII* that in each lesson, a new *objet a* is held up to the students by the teacher: the signifier whose function is to be understood or learnt. For most educators, in parading this signifier they take on the mirror image of the ideal-ego, the Imaginary figure that the Other of the student could become if only they pursue the object. This mirror image is a demand to be seen as the holder of the signifier of lack, the S.s.S., the master. Teaching becomes a sales pitch, as in the space of the classroom this object proffered as desirable by the teacher and (hopefully) pursued by the student. But what happens in the voyage of the letter is that students do not receive the object being offered, but rather receive something else, something Real that we cannot ever formulate. This leaves the Symbolic of education, both in terms of curriculum and of pedagogy, in tatters, so that the teacher is left with only desire and jouissance.

Lacan knows all of this in his own formulation of desire. Following on from 'The Purloined Letter', Lacan notes in his essay 'The Instance of the Letter in the Unconscious' that desire 'envelops the pleasure of knowing and of dominating in jouissance' (E, p. 431). The classroom's structure of desire offers a certain form of jouissance and it is far from what conventional and 'progressive' accounts of teaching and learning represent. In *Seminar VIII*, a claim about 'the goal of teaching' (VIII, p. 251) is made: to avoid the intensification of understanding by the students in 'uselessly multiplying in order to provide superficial analogies and intellectual aids' (p. 251). Lacan resists the drive that teachers feel in their identification with the figure of the teacher, to ceaselessly redescribe and represent the issue at the heart of the lesson so to keep making the *objet a* desirable for the Other. In Lacan's implicit redescription, there is a dimension of desire addressed that replays the logic of fort-da. The teacher withholds the object through the detour, anticipating the reveal that can never quite happen, partly because the object is always, in some deep-seated sense, unknowable in its 'essence'. The jouissance of teaching is in the withholding and in the partial reveal, although for the students it may be less certain.

Lacan is enacting an important doubling in his teaching that is worth consideration. Though he still *initially* takes on the mantle of the master by assuming the position of the teacher, he rejects the demand to be heard and understood by his students knowing its impossibility. He still has things he desires to teach but does not construct them into clear signifiers to be desired by the students. He visibly enjoys the act of teaching, but always with an auto-critique, a meta-theatricality, an irony: features that in tragic theatre are expressed through the chorus function, through plays within plays, through the figure of the fool. Ultimately, Lacan seems to find a way of being and enjoying being a teacher *within* the inescapable

Symbolic order of education *qua* classroom, whilst rejecting the Symbolic law that the space engenders. As Richards underscores, 'Lacan himself says in the unpublished seminar R.S.I.: "say any old rubbish; it will always touch the truth"' (2024, p. 69). We might move towards the close of this book with some words on words, then.

The Signifier and La Langue

Much of what we have explored in this chapter has circled around the notion of talking, speaking, even singing, whether on stage or in the classroom. The 'signifier is the apparatus of jouissance' (Miller, 2019b, p. 53), the very vessel through which our jouissance is made possible. To condense these ideas, we turn again to Barthes:

> Imagine that I am a teacher: I speak, endlessly, in front of and for someone who remains silent. I am the person who says I (the detours of one, we or impersonal sentence make no difference), I am the person who, under cover of setting out a body of knowledge, puts out a discourse, never knowing how that discourse is being received and thus forever forbidden the reassurance of a definitive image—even if offensive—which would constitute me. (Barthes, 1977a, p. 194)

Barthes suggests in his presentation of teaching in *Writers, Intellectuals, Teachers,* an essay that makes regular reference to Lacan's work, that the teacher is always putting discourse out into the little world of the classroom, delivering letters to the students. Barthes too recognizes the detour of the letter, and the impossibility of what he consciously intends to be heard being heard. What teachers in all forms demand is that their letter arrive at a destination they can determine, that is, that their voice is heard by the Other as it was intended. We know, of course, that it will always be received by the Other. That does not mean it is received in the way that is intended, that one even knows what is intended, or that the Other can be centred in an individual subject. What we wonder here is whether this process might still be enjoyable even if we are not being heard.

As we have raised in previous chapters, teaching is embroiled in the signifier in a way that no other profession can be: "professional talkers" as we once heard them called. From its earliest stages, the focus on language acquisition, reading and writing, literacy levels, and moves from simple to complex vocabulary, centre the signifier *qua* signifier. Teachers in the classroom talk *ad infinitum*, from a greeting at the door, to starting the lesson, to working through a question, to reading an extract, to doling out disciplinary statements, to going off on tangents about their partner, and so on. The 'jouissance of blahblahblah' (Miller, 2019b, p. 64) is present in most teachers: one of us remembers lessons we have taught where we introduce the introduction to a new text, say, *A Streetcar Named Desire*, only to then introduce it, then to actually begin it, which involves the reading aloud of it. Even when the text is in full swing a few scenes (and lessons) down the road, the voice of the students might echo around the room whilst they scream "STEEELLLLLAHHHH", but the teacher interjects, analyses, supplements the voices of the students. Even if the lesson is driven by student voices, classroom discussions, 'oral strategies', the students are to work through a signifier instigated by the teacher. 'Discuss the reasons you think Stella goes back to Stanley at the end of this scene, making reference to quotes and features in the scene in your groups.' The signifier as signifier is in many ways what teaching is, as says Lacan: 'There is no way of following me without passing through my signifiers, but to pass through signifiers involves the feeling of alienation that incites them to seek' (XI, p. 217). The student must pass through the teacher's signifiers, signifiers that do not belong to the teacher but are found in the locus of the big Other through the Symbolic of education. This is quotidian in the classroom, as students are often required to not only learn to repeat the signifiers of the teacher, which of course are repetitions of the curriculum, but so too must they pass through the acceptance of the teacher: 'a good response', 'wrong answer', 'could you expand on that for me?', 'tell your partner', and so forth … These signifiers determine the following of the teacher (an omnipresent assessment of student by teacher), but they also alienate and split the student. Nevertheless, for the purpose of this chapter, we maintain that the signifier as part of teaching is where the possibility of modes of enjoyment arise. As Lacan says, 'The signifier is the cause of *jouissance*' (XX, p. 24).

The signifier as carried by the voice, the central feature of the very process of analysis in the clinic, is also a feature of desire for Lacan. It is curious that, whilst 'Lacan devoted a significant part of Seminar XI to the scopic object, there is not a comparable development of the object voice in Lacan's teaching' (Millar, 2021, p. 78). This is curious in the sense that Lacan, as we have made clear, spends much time exploring his own enjoyment as a teacher. Nevertheless, the voice is one of the key partial objects of desire for Lacan that circles round the 'invocatory drive' (XI, p. 118).

Put simply, the voice holds pleasure for the listener, empirically clear in the rise of ASMR, or as Millar (2021) explores, the erotic pleasure of interacting with the disembodied voice of an AI in Jonze's 2013 film *Her*. If we are to find enjoyment in a classroom, then, it is likely in the voice that we will find it. We have discussed the gaze at play in the classroom in earlier chapters, but ultimately it is hearing the voice of the teacher has the potential of pleasure, maybe something with the potential of jouissance, though invariably dutiful obedience to the Symbolic order of education may deflect this.

Returning to Barthes's observations of the classroom and the enunciations of the teacher, he notes the conformity of the teacher to the Law. As indicated, this Law is discussed by Lacan in *Seminar VII* and elsewhere, a master signifier of the father, the name of the father (*nom du pere*) as Lacan calls it. As we discussed in Chap. 1, there is such a law of the classroom too, the demand to educate no matter what. To speak in a teaching space is to play a part in the 'theatre of speech' (Barthes, 1977a, p. 192), to repeat the lines that are demanded when one enters the subjectivating space of the classroom. If one is to seek new forms of jouissance, one must 'subvert the Law' (p. 192), that is, escape the jouissance of the imperative to educate. If we think about this in terms of the voice and the signifiers that spring forth, 'the teacher would have to undermine voice delivery, word speed, and rhythm to the point of *another* [an Other] intelligibility' (p. 192). Put differently, it is only when the voice is 'a-phonic' (Miller, 2007, p. 139), taking on the substanceless form of the *objet a* that '*falls from the body*' (Millar, 2021, p. 79) that the enjoyment sought is made available. Voice operates between Symbolic and Real; there's pleasure in voice independent of signifier (as in ululation and such like). It must resist or exceed signification if it is to be pleasurable or enjoyable, something that presents a paradoxical predicament in the classroom. As we said, the classroom is the house of the signifier *qua* signifier; it is the very place where the mode of signification unfurls. A typical pedagogical encounter revolves around 'learning a new term'. In teaching the term 'synechdoche' for example, one might give a definition, 'where the part represents the whole', an example, 'my new wheels', and a similar term, 'a form of metaphor'. What has happened in this simple encounter, in the chain of signifiers from term to definition to example to synonym, reinforces the Symbolic of the educational order. So, like with tragic laughter, how does one seek to reformulate such an activity as aphonia?

Think of a child learning to speak, what Lacan refers to as *lalangue*. A child seen at 17 months, stringing together sounds for the first few times, learning to say (not identify) a word like 'flower', is a sort of enjoyment we rarely consider. Children sometimes sneak downstairs from bed to sit on the stairs just to listen to their parents talking to their friends, even if they cannot understand the words being exchanged. It is the jouissance of the signifier, not the sign—an absolute meaning of a linguistic unit, or of the signifying chain—what the signifier might relate to. It is rather the signifier with its inherently arbitrary referent, a unit that stands on its own as inherently enjoyable rather than being redeployed for the Symbolic function of education as pedagogical. As such, it is not about understanding, but only saying and listening though not necessarily understanding.

Lacan thinks this enjoyment through James Joyce (E, XX, XXIII). Joyce arguably uses the signifier not to create understanding or to command meaning, but rather because of the enjoyment of the signifier. As Thurston notes:

> This kind of language would correspond to what Lacan writes as *lalangue*—speech embodying an infantile *la-la*—or *jouis-sens*, the coalescence of meaning and enjoyment. The crucial point is that, for Lacan, language 'normally' prohibits jouissance ... *Jouis-sens*—or Joycesense, as we should perhaps write it—is thus above all ... something naughty: in other words, both nothing-at-all, founded on naught or the void, and a childish or impish defiance of paternal authority. (Thurston, 2004, p. 112)

We might desire to understand Joyce, of course, but the mode of his prose inhibits this desire and jouissance. *Finnegan's Wake* is Lacan's oft-used example throughout Seminar XXIII, but we might turn to *Ulysses* not least because, alongside *A Portrait of the Artist as a Young Man*, it is a 'forensic analysis' of 'elite education' (Platt, 2021, p. 89) and its ultimate failure to redeem its subjects. Joyce even gives an example of the pedagogic scene in the chapter 'Nestor' in *Ulysses,* and we might find traces of the aphonic mode in not just the prose style but the actions of the characters. In it we see Stephen Dedalus attempt to teach a history lesson. 'Do you understand now?' (1922, p. 43) he repeats throughout the lesson, demanding the pedagogic relation be complete. Stephen abandons history halfway through to teach poetry, perhaps a sign of following his own desires in the classroom rather than external demands. But it goes further than this, for what we see is

> Stephen is a cog in a wheel and his lesson a waste of time. A fragmented mess in terms of content, in style it is characterized by meaningless tests of memory, a poor joke which his pupils fail to get and an incomprehensible riddle. (Platt, 2021, p. 91)

Not only does Stepehen prove to be a prop in the Symbolic order of education, but he also moves into aphonia, an incomprehensible riddle of his own that students cannot follow. The very prose of the novel is of course a both formal and linguistic presentation of the 'blahblahblah'. Joyce's puns, allusions, homonyms, riddles, malapropisms, narrative distortion, tantalise a necessity to understand but equally deny total interpretation. In any line, the 'seaspawn and seawrack, the nearing tide, that rusty boot. Snotgreen, bluesilver, rust: coloured signs' (Joyce, 1922, p. 64), Joyce has pushed beyond the pedagogical mode and the demand for an understanding of the signifier. The signifiers here are, in a way, without purpose, and to revel in them is to enjoy the way they 'fit together, combine, and concertina' (XX, p. 37). They are like that of a patient in a session of analysis who starts unconsciously weaving together the signifiers of their dreams, their traumas, and their desires. But we must remember that jouissance is not teaching Joyce; this is not an attempt to pedagogize Joyce by seeking to understand the signifiers he uses. This would be to impose non-lack on the signifier, to make it the act of the insertion. It is the reading, speaking, hearing Joyce that is imbued with jouissance. The 'blahblahblah' of speaking 'means that it is not a question of communication … [Only that] there is a body who speaks' (Miller, 2019b, p. 73). In the classroom, if we speak, listen, not engage in a pedagogical relation, but rather in the play of the signifier, there is a jouissance to be found. It is not something we would call educational, but we might find it enjoyable. We must learn to enjoy the signifier in the relation between teacher and student, not for the utility that the signifier brings, but merely for the signifier itself.

Early Derrida's key themes return again and again to this post-Saussurian analysis of the sign and its instability, the play and temporality of signification, the deferral of meaning, spacing, decentred textual being, the idea of writing as system or technology as against the idea of the voice as guarantee of presence: all of these key themes chime with the Lacanian thinking of the signifier, whereby meanings are mobile, dynamic, always susceptible to 'play', above and beyond any rational intentionality. On the other hand, curriculized pedagogy must unconsciously set strict if invisible limits to the linguistic field, limiting speaking, reading and responding to attempt to regulate them within the institutional framework of schooling. Derrida's linked ideas of dispersal, trace and dissemination, for instance, render language and textual material (the curriculum, in effect) a mobile field of 'play', potentially open to more fluid conceptions and practices of meaning that may suggest a drastic critique of the everyday pedagogy, and that certainly highlight a difficulty for straight pedagogic action (liberal or formal).

Derrida's position emphasises differences and 'play' in discourse:

> a system in which the central signified, the original or transcendental signified, is never absolutely present outside a system of differences. The absence of the transcendental signified extends the domain and the play of signification infinitely. (Derrida, 1978, p. 280)

Here the uncertain centre surely puts into question the holding principles of textual study further problematized by Derrida's insistence on the infinite extension of the 'domain' of signification and its endless 'play'. While liberal pedagogic practices encourage the personal engagement and response of students that 'response' is always already constrained in an invisible forcefield of legitimated meanings or response positions. The curriculized pedagogic dream of 'the textbook' is always problematized by the exclusion in Derrida of totalization:

> If totalization no longer has any meaning, it is not because the infiniteness of a field cannot be covered by a finite glance or a finite discourse, but because the nature of the field—that is, language and a finite language—excludes totalization. This field is in effect that of *play*, that is to say a field of infinite substitutions only because it is finite, that is to say, because instead of being an inexhaustible field, as in the classical hypothesis, instead of being too large, there is something missing from it: a center which arrests and grounds the play of substitutions. One could say—rigorously using that word whose scandalous signification is always obliterated in French—that this movement of play, permitted by the lack or absence of a center of origin, is the movement of *supplementarity*. One cannot determine the center and exhaust totalization because the sign which replaces the center, which supplements it, taking the center's place in its absence—this sign is added, occurs as a surplus, as a *supplement*. The movement of signification adds something, which results in the fact that there is always more, but this addition is a floating one because it comes to perform a vicarious function, to supplement a lack on the part of the signified. (Derrida, 1978, p. 289)

Rootless supplementarity—as constant movement of the signifier—indicates a paradoxical logic enforcing acknowledgement of the intertextuality of meanings and meaning systems. According to the Derridean position, not only are meanings subject to endless play and endless deferment, meanings are also always dependent on something else the text in question cannot supply. The signifier is always reaching beyond itself: 'The overabundance of the signifier, its supplementary character, is thus the result of a finitude, that is to say, the result of a lack which must be supplemented' (Derrida, 1978, p. 290).

Textual meanings are constrained, but play and supplementarity emphasise the enormous significance of institutional frameworks for meaning. In the meantime, we may ask what happens if we put 'play' (or aphonia, or lalangue) into play? Interpretations and meanings must then be seen as forces at work in the management of meanings, required to supplement the restless interplay of infinitude and lack (finitude) in texts. What's more

> Communication presupposes subjects (whose identity and presence are constituted before the signifying operation) and objects (signified concepts, a thought meaning that the passage of communication will have neither to constitute, nor, by all rights, to transform). *A* communicates *B* to *C*. (Derrida, 1978, p. 293)

Isn't Derrida's interrogation and suspicion of communication another version of the phenomenology of objet a? The paradox of supplementarity and play is what makes signification in itself an uncanny business. The centring of linguistic events (texts?)—according to principles such as authorship and meaning—must always depend on something that comes from outside, that is imposed, as it were, by contexts, discourses and social practices that hold the Symbolic order in a kind of stability.

Derrida's thesis reminds us of the anchoring of meaning by Western metaphysics, an extended version of what the lawyer in *Bartleby* ... refers to as 'common usage', amounting to the freighting of language with a politics of meaning:

> Now, 'everyday language' is not innocent or neutral. It is the language of Western metaphysics, and it carries with it not only a considerable number of presuppositions of all types, but also presuppositions inseparable from metaphysics, which ... are knotted into a system. (Derrida, 1987, p. 19)

Systems of thought constitute the limits for the possibilities of discourse. It is not too much of a leap to relate this idea to the domination of the specific discourse of teaching by oppositions that have institutional power and that are carried forward in the construction of professional identity, in the authorized practices, in examination syllabuses, in established publications, in national curricula as well as in the casual professional exchanges of teachers. At the same time, the extended Derridean account of language (grammatology) includes the possibility of deconstruction, whereby habitual oppositional and complementary concepts are subject to a degree of play. This means that while the Symbolic order cannot be overthrown by any abrupt radical revolution in thinking, it must always be subject to a degree of play. Our contention here is that it is possible, as a mundane teacher, to allow for and engage in play to activate a jouissance that is not necessarily and always identical with the jouissance of the model teacher.

Hysterical Pedagogy

Derrida's often more than faintly Lacanian 'reminders' of generally unrevealed features of language and textuality—spacing, supplementarity, the trace, and so on—offer a different set of ideas for rethinking the meaning of practices in teaching, including all those ameliorative and salvific embedded ideas that we have referred to. But perhaps we might find resonance in the clinical work of Lacan and this play of signification that Derrida dwelt on. Such movements are best characterised in the Lacanian field as the voice of the hysteric. There is a common usage of hysteric/hysteria that neither we nor Lacan subscribes to, as discussed in the following paragraph. But the reason we bring up the hysteric is because of their dominant mode as a talker, and one who's meaning needs constant interrogation due the way the unconscious plays with the talking. Like Joyce's writing or Derrida's deconstruction, the hysteric is another figure of the blahblahblah that we might find some traces of Other enjoyment.

Hysteria was eliminated from the DSM in 1952, spelling the end of the term's usage for diagnosis beyond the dwindling field of psychoanalysis. In Freud and Breur's 1895 *Studies on Hysteria* (SE II), Anna O famously coined the term 'the talking cure' to describe the process that would come to be known as psychoanalysis. In Freud's case study 'Dora' (SE VII), Dora presented with catarrh and a cough that had no identifiable physiological source. Believing her symptoms were produced by an unconscious fantasy that involved her father and his illicit lover Frau K, Freud traced the love affair that Dora stated she was repelled by but unconsciously acted in ways that seemed to enable the relationship. Alongside a sexual assault by Herr K, the husband of Frau K, she forged an unlikely alliance with Frau K that raised questions concerning sex and sexuality previously repressed in her bourgeois family circle. Freud's greatest misstep was to claim and then assert that Dora's unconscious desire was directed towards Herr K, an assertion that prompted her to cease her analysis. Lacan's re-evaluation of the case challenges Dora's unconscious fantasy, believing the symptoms were a 'means of questioning her femininity' (Cavasola, 2015, p. 1) as opposed to an expression of desire for Herr K.

The Lacanian re-evaluation of Dora's case is structural rather than personal, and thus offers an interesting position that we might find useful for rethinking the enjoyment of the teacher. Dora's position as a young woman in the middle of a family affair ultimately raised questions about women and sexuality that she struggled to process, Lacan says (E, p. 179), resulting in not only her symptoms, but also an inability to piece together her own sense of self. Put differently, the place she held within a very particular Symbolic order (the nineteenth century bourgeois family) resulted in a certain set of symptoms, including a mode of speech. This speech was a 'functional fragmentation' (Webster, 2015, p. 1); listening to her was like 'trying to navigate an unnavigable river' (p. 1), yet this is not to say that it is garbled or incoherent. The hysterical voice is, as Webster says, characterised by the 'intense intricacy of what comes to be said', 'maddening, mystifying and magical' (2024, p. 68). Hysterics are in the mode of production of new grammars, images, metaphors (Gherovici, 2014, p. 54) as they unconsciously succumb to, as Lacan says, the 'birth of truth in speech' (E, p. 212). They are not figures of clarity; we are always confronted in the speaking riddle of hysteric's demand to produce the new (p. 64). But they are, as Lacan makes clear, the only ones who can produce something new—whether that be the creation of the talking cure or of a great work of art (p. 51-52), or maybe a lesson ... The student might well be tantalised by the poetry of the hysteric forever attempting to unravel their riddles, but not learning from them, or certainly not being taught anything. Like the radical alterity of Joyce and Derrida, the aphonic, the mode of the blahblahblah, there are 'kernel[s] of trauma' (p. 68) in what is said, or perhaps fragments of the Real that can be parsed. This is not an appeal to truth, however, something troubled by our account of knowledge in Chap. 4. Instead it is a mode of speech that denies the easy enveloping into the neatness of Symbolic order, but at the same time one that speaks of the very Symbolic that engenders it. Again, this not saying what is oppressive about the situation to the students. This appeals to a pedagogical coherence that the hysteric could never be slotted into.

Webster (2023, p. 914) identifies Lacan as a hysterical teacher, one who wonders around on stage making wild free-associations. This puts the audience in the position of analyst, listener to the hysteric, as the one who seeks to understand, but not to receive passively. It also ensures they are prone to failure, lacking in the truth, unable to reach any finally revelatory discovery. Only the hysteric does that. This is essential for enjoyment, as Webster makes clear that the hysterical question of desire opens the possibility of a '*jouissance* as Other, as an excess, not simply the filling of lack' (p. 928). As such, the enjoyment that is not the attendance to the Other's lack, is only to be obtained in the hysterical mode of the teacher, a feminine mode (p. 928), an acceptance of the teacher as questioning their place as a subject and interrogating the nature of their desire. What does such excess of enjoyment look like for the teacher? It must spill beyond the master, must leak through the confines of the Symbolic. It cannot be simply part of the educational Symbolic order, which means, of course, to modify the desire to educate in pursuit of an Other form of enjoyment.

This said, in *Monsieur Lazhar*, mentioned in Chap. 3, the film begins with the suicide of a teacher, her body discovered by two of her students. The whole class traumatised, it is clear that there is no escape from the repression of trauma for the class and a consequent hystericization of the classroom occurs. Against the grain of pedagogic norms, Lazhar brings that trauma into the classroom, speaking of it and asking that students do too. Students respond by acting violently, or musing on the nature of death; they enter the tragic mode rather than automatically resuming the push for positivity. A therapist visits the class and demands Lazhar remains outside the classroom to 'separate psychotherapy from pedagogy', but of course this only serves to punctuate the notion that the dialectical relationship between these two things demands that they cannot be pulled apart. Other students reveal suicide in their own family, with memories of relatives escaping political persecution as indeed Lazhar is himself. It is these experiences that students are made to repress in their educational experience that values progress above the opening of the unconscious, or to paraphrase Freud, pursue knowledge over breaking down psychic resistance. Like the hysteric, the teacher does not choose what to consciously bring into teaching. The unconscious chooses for us. As one student neatly observes, 'Everyone thinks we're traumatised, but it is the adults who are.' We bring this film up not to encourage teachers to discuss trauma in their lessons, something that would inevitably be folded back into an educational Symbolic narrative anyway. Rather, it is to offer images of the blahblahblah, the hysterical speaker, the teacher not committed to the demand to educate. This blahblahblah of Lazhar is what allowed for the unconscious to enter.

In this manner, as knowledge does little to help hysteria, a hysterical pedagogy accommodates the 'mismatch between knowledge and desire, or sense and nonsense … By tolerating paradoxes, exploring conflicting tendencies, and being aware of inconsistencies in … discourse' (Grose, 2016, p. xxix). This is not simply a move to accept student dialogue or 'listen to their voice'—both things that are problematic for psychoanalytic thinking—but rather suggests an attunement to the unconscious messiness of the transferential space of the classroom, a space dominated by the movement of signifiers from teacher to student and back again. We might see how Lacan refused to curricularise his teaching: it rarely stayed on the theme he started with, and would push to new topics each session. But by the same token, it was not ever a coherent body of knowledge to be obtained or learned. It was a 'fantasia on a theme', a play on a structure, that denied the possibility of being fully heard, enjoyed mostly by Lacan himself in his position on the stage. Such a figure cannot be seen as holding a signifier of lack; is he holding anything at all? Hysterical pedagogy always seeks the new, never settles on what has been supposedly learned or unlearned.

We should also not that the hysteric is in continual defiance of the master, but do not wish to confuse this with the veiling of the figure of the teacher found in critical pedagogy. Defiance of the master is at the level of the big Other, not of quotidian classroom law. To refuse to take the register or to teach a topic you would prefer is pleasurable in its defiance, but a rejection of the logic of progress and its upwards curve (including towards consciousness) is necessary to seek hysterical jouissance. It is necessarily an act of the death drive. We cannot speak it here, but we wonder what would hystericized pedagogy have to say … what would we have to *hear,* that would be so Other to that which we hear in the classroom day to day? How would the teacher who speaks respond to the symbolic order into which they were thrown? We are faced with Real of education—an intolerable dimension of the supposedly benign and inherently redemptive.

A hysterical pedagogue is one who arouses the desire of the Other and leaves it unsatisfied. The educational myth of wholeness is defied by such logic, but it calls for an engagement with the student as Other as opposed to the 'educational Other' (Fink, 1999, p. 33) that is upheld in most discourse around even liberatory pedagogy. Hysterical pedagogy is not a reenactment of the educational demand to educate, but an opening of oneself to the Other in the space of the classroom—it is 'identification at the level of desire' (VIII, p. 355), it is a riddled search for the new with no promise of wholeness or betterment. We find this made more transparent in Seminar X where Lacan outlines some structures for pedagogy, favouring what he calls 'the function of the key (X, p. 21). Of course, this is a signifier of possessing the ability to unlock the students' knowledge, but the Lacanian irony remains in the figure of the teacher as the key holder who never has to give that key over. It remains firmly in the hand of the teacher with no guarantee it can be enunciated. Teaching becomes hystericized in the search for the key to meaning, but one that is not given over to the students. Perhaps now we might ironically understand more clearly what Lacan meant by his statement 'I explain nothing' (XVI, p. 139). It is fine to masquerade the position of the key holder, so long as the key is never used to try to and unlock anything.

Closing Remarks

To return to the question from the opening of this book, What is a Lacanian teacher? Lacan's claim that the death drive is a mode of radical alterity, a 'strain of a totally different nature' (XVI, p. 95), and as such opens the possibility of something very different going on in classrooms, but not something that could in any Symbolically appropriate way be called education. But the space of education, its stage, its impossible relationality, its desires, its fantasies, are all ready to be enjoyed in divergent ways. We have, in different ways, asserted that though the classroom may be an unknowable and thoroughly unredemptive sort of place, that does not mean there are not things worth examining, traversing and enacting there. It is simply that those things might not be what we (and others) would call educational.

As raised at the start of the chapter, there are numerous forms of jouissance available for the teacher. It has been made clear that teachers are already enjoying themselves, though usually this is in the relation of non-lack they believe to have with the students they teach via the big Other 'education'. This engenders other forms of sadomasochistic jouissance to take place in the necessitation of a pedagogised mode of being. And yet, there are Other forms of jouissance made possible through a reorienting and reimagining of the teacher in the classroom as the Lacanian teacher. This tragic figure who accepts their death—that is, the end of education—plays with the voice of the hysteric, seeks not for meaning but only for speaking, opens such possibilities.

To accept the end of education, the illusion of its salvific fantasy and its ameliorative essence means giving up on its ontotheological pretensions to both individual and collective redemption. As Julie Reshe gleefully notes, there is no salvation in jouissance:

> In Lacan's theory, since jouissance presupposes both pleasure and pain it is "beyond the pleasure principle" (Lacan 1973/1994, p. 184). The logic of conceptualisation of jouissance mirrors Freudian death drive; both are self-subversive and work contrary to the attainment of the pleasure and balance. Jouissance functions as a painful principle, for Lacan, "jouissance … is suffering" (Lacan 1959–1960/1992, p. 184). This makes jouissance "the path towards death" (Lacan 1969–70/1991, p. 17). (Reshe, 2023, p. 37)

Jouissance, we might say, is an-archic, without founding principle, without telos, but at the same time, as Catherine Malabou (2023) claims, 'anarchist being' is the question of life as survival, perhaps an urgent matter in present times. For Malabou, another vision arises from the serious contemplation of the death-drive, free from the redemptive telos of education's vast apparatus:

> In the solitude of vast Siberian steppes, under the pale gleam of the winter sun, watching animals help each other, Kropotkin concluded that mutual aid deposes natural selection from its status as principle. Mutual aid is the social response of nature, and is thus a key example of the death drive turning back on itself. (Malabou, 2023, p. 219)

Could not this image capture something of 'what makes life worth living' available to the destituted Lacanian teacher? For the teacher aspiring to an anarchic mode of being that is not identical with the big other's law of the classroom?

References

Others

Barthes, R. (1977a). Writers, Intellectuals, Professors. In *Image, Music, Text* (pp. 190–215). Fontana Press.
Barthes, R. (1977b). *Roland Barthes* (R. Howard, Trans.). Hill and Wang.
Beckett, S. (1983). *Worstward Ho.* Calder.
Benjamin, W. (1970). *Illuminations.* Johnathan Cape.
Bergmark, U., Lundström, S., Manderstedt, L., & Palo, A. (2018). Why Become a Teacher? Student Teachers' Perceptions of the Teaching Profession and Motives for Career Choice. *European Journal of Teacher Education, 41*(3), 266–281.
Brecht, B. (1964 [2013]). *The Resistible Rise of Arturo Ui.* Methuen Drama.
Brecht, B. (2018). *Brecht on Theatre* (M. Silberman, et al., Eds.). Bloomsbury Publishing.
Britzman, D. (1991). *Practice Makes Practice: A Critical Study of Learning to Teach.* SUNY Press.
Britzman, D. (2015). *A Psychoanalyst in the Classroom.* SUNY Press.
Cavasola, R. (2015). A Reading of Contemporary Hysteria from Lacan's teachings. *European Journal of Psychoanalysis, 2*(1). (online, n. pg).
Cioran, E.M. (2018 [1975]). *A Short History of Decay.* Penguin Books.
Clarke, M. (2023). The Subordination of Teacher Identity: Ethical Risks and Potential Lines of Flight. *Teachers & Teaching Theory & Practice, 29*(3), 241–258.
Clarke, M., & Phelan, A. (2017). *Teacher Education and the Political: The Power of Negative Thinking* (1st ed.). Routledge.
Copjec, J. (2015). *Read My Desire. Lacan Against the Historicists.* Verso.
Critchley, S. (1999). Comedy and Finitude: Displacing the Tragic-Heroic Paradigm in Philosophy and Psychoanalysis. *Constellations, 6*, 108–122.
Derrida, J. (1978). Structure, Sign and Play in the Discourse of the Human Sciences. In *Writing and Difference.* Routledge and Kegan Paul.
Derrida, J. (1987). *Positions* (A. Bass & C. Norris, Eds.). Continuum.
Derrida, J. (1998). *Resistances of Psychoanalysis.* Stanford University Press.
DfE. (2022). *Political Impartiality in Schools.* https://www.gov.uk/government/publications/political-impartiality-in-schools/political-impartiality-in-schools
Donald, J. (1992). *Sentimental Education: School, Popular Culture and the Regulation of Liberty.* Verso.
Eagleton, T. (1986). *William Shakespeare.* Blackwell.
Ellis, V. (Ed.). (2024). *Teacher Education in Crisis: The State, the Market and the Universities in England.* Bloomsbury Academic.
Faladé, S. (1996). Penia et Poros, du récit mythique à l'événement historique. In R. Toumson (Ed.), *Portulan: Négritude, Antillanité, Créolité. Revue des Caraïbes et des Amériques noires* (pp. 139–147). Jutta Hepke.

Felman, S. (1982). Psychoanalysis and Education: Teaching Terminable and Interminable. *Yale French Studies, 63*, 21–44.
Fink, B. (1999). *A Clinical Introduction to Lacanian Psychoanalysis: Theory and Technique*. Harvard University Press.
Flores, M. A. (2023). Teacher Education in Times of Crisis: Enhancing or Deprofessionalising the Teaching Profession? *European Journal of Teacher Education, 46*(2), 199–202.
Frimberger, K. (2022). "Cultivating the Art of Living": The Pleasures of Bertolt Brecht's Philosophising Theatre Pedagogy. *Studies in Philosophy and Education 41*(6): 653–668.
Gherovici, P. (2014). Where Have the Hysterics Gone?: Lacan's Reinvention of Hysteria. *ESC, 40*(1), 47–70.
Gorard, S., Maria Ventista, O., Morris, R., & See, B. H. (2023). Who Wants to be a Teacher? Findings from a Survey of Undergraduates in England. *Educational Studies, 49*(6), 914–936. https://doi.org/10.1080/03055698.2021.1915751
Grose, A. (Ed.). (2016). *Hysteria Today*. Routledge.
Heidegger, M. (1977). *The Question Concerning Technology, and Other Essays*. New York: Harper & Row.
Heron, J., & Johnson, N. (2020). Beckettian Pedagogies: Learning through Samuel Beckett. *Journal of Beckett Studies, 29*(1), 42–62.
Hunter, I. (1994). *Rethinking the School: Subjectivity, Bureaucracy, Criticism* (1st ed.). Routledge.
Jameson, F. (1998). *Brecht and Method*. Verso.
Joyce, J. (1922). *Ulysses*. Penguin Classics.
Lortie, D. (1975). *Schoolteacher: A Sociological Study*. University of Chicago Press.
Malabou, C. (2010). *Plasticity at the Dusk of Writing*. Columbia University Press.
Malabou, C. (2012). *Ontology of the Accident: An Essay on Destructive Plasticity* (C. P. T. Shread, Ed.). Polity.
Malabou, C. (2023). *Stop Thief! Anarchism and Philosophy*. Polity.
Millar, I. (2021). *The Psychoanalysis of Artificial Intelligence*. Palgrave.
Miller, J.-A. (2007). Jacques Lacan and the Voice. In V. Voruz & B. Wolf (Eds.), *The Later Lacan: An Introduction* (pp. 137–146). SUNY.
Miller, J.-A. (2019a). The Turin Theory of the Subject of the School. In *The Real and the Social Bond. Psychoanalytic Notebooks, 33*. London Society of the NLS.
Miller, J.-A. (2019b). Paradigms of Jouissance. In *Paradigms. Psychoanalytic Notebooks, 34*. London Society of the NLS.
Nietzsche, F. (1872 [2008]). *The Birth of Tragedy: Out of the Spirit of Music*. Oxford University Press.
O'Donnell, A. (2014). Reflections on Beckett and Education. *Journal of Philosophy of Education, 48*, 260–275.
Peim, N. (2016). Philosophy, Tragedy, and Education: Thinking After Nihilism. *Other Education, 5*(2), 87–107.
Peim, N. (2022). *Rethinking the Politics of Education*. Routledge.

Platt, L. (2021). *James Joyce and Education. Schooling and the Social Imaginary in the Modernist Novel.* Routledge.

Poole, A. (2023). *Teachers' and Leaders' Lived Experiences of the School Inspection System in England. A Case Study of Two Secondary Schools Serving Disadvantaged Communities.* University of Sussex. Thesis. https://hdl.handle.net/10779/uos.24278836.v1

Reay, D. (2022). The Slide to Authoritarianism in English Schools. *The Forum, 64*(3), 126–139.

Reshe, J. (2023). *Negative Psychoanalysis for the Living Dead. Philosophical Pessimism and the Death Drive.* Palgrave Macmillan.

Richards, S. (2023). A Lesson for the World: Solange Faladé's Anti-colonial Multiracialism. *Modern & Contemporary France, 31*(4), 435–450.

Richards, S. (2024). 'I Am a Clown': Lacan's Difficult Literary Dandyism. *Paragraph, 47*(1), 59–73.

Said, E. W. (2003). *Orientalism.* Penguin Classics.

Schutz, P. A., Crowder, K. C., & White, V. E. (2001). The Development of a Goal to Become a Teacher. *Journal of Educational Psychology, 93*(2), 299–230.

Stahl, G., Keddie, A., & Adams, B. (2022). The Manosphere Goes to School: Problematizing Incel Surveillance through Affective Boyhood. *Educational Philosophy and Theory, 55*(3), 366–378.

Stock, N. (2020). Paradise Shall Remain Lost: Readdressing Deschooling Through a Miltonian Lens. *Other Education, 9*(2), 3–20.

Swales, S. (2023). Depression Reconsidered. In D. Hook & S. Vanheule (Eds.), *Lacan on Depression and Melancholia* (pp. 20–28). Routledge.

Thurston, L. (2004). *James Joyce and the Problem of Psychoanalysis.* Cambridge University Press.

Vernant, Jean-Pierre & Vidal-Naquet, Pierre. (1990). *Myth and Tragedy in Ancient Greece.* Zone Books.

Webster, J. (2015). Begin Again: Hysteria as Forgetting, Repetition, and Atonement. *European Journal of Psychoanalysis, 2*(1).

Webster, J. (2022). *Disorganization and Sex.* Divided.

Webster, J. (2023). The Most Hysterical Psychoanalyst. *Journal of the American Psychoanalytic Association, 71*(5), 907–931.

Webster, J. (2024). How Not to Kill a Hysteric. In A. Taheri, C. Vanderwees, & R. Naderi (Eds.), *Philosophy After Lacan: Politics, Science, and Art* (1st ed., pp. 68–82). Routledge.

Wright, E. (1989). *Postmodern Brecht. A Re-Presentation.* Routledge.

Žižek, S. (2009). *The Parallax View.* MIT Press.

Zupančič, A. (2003). Ethics and Tragedy in Lacan. In J.-M. Rabaté (Ed.), *The Cambridge Companion to Lacan* (pp. 173–190). Cambridge University Press.

Zupančič, A. (2008). *The Odd One In: On Comedy.* MIT Press.

Glossary

Alienation For Lacan alienation is the inescapable condition of the subject. The subject is fundamentally split and, rather curiously, barred from itself. The subject is alienated from its own desire that remains both obscure to it and restlessly beyond the management of its conscious control. The subject is alienated in and through language where the big Other appears as the other within, the subject being subjected to semantic and syntactic motility. Lacan deploys the Rimbaud quote: 'I is an other' (E, p. 23) to emphasize the alienation of the Imaginary order.

Anxiety We experience anxiety beyond the Symbolic and Imaginary order (like jouissance). It is the feeling of coming too close to the Real that cannot be put into language. Anxiety has the same structure as fantasy, as it is predicated on the subject's interaction with the object of their desire. A teacher who encounters a lack of acceptance by a student they believed to be idolised by would thus be an experience of anxiety.

Big Other See Other/other.

Borromean knot Lacan's interest in topology is reflected in his invocation of the Borromean knot, a three-ringed knot that becomes unravelled if any one of its rings is severed. There is an obvious parallel between the Borromean knot and Lacan's three-way ontology comprising the Symbolic, the Imaginary and the Real, dimensions of being that intersect, overlap and that are mutually dependent. In psychoanalytic

© The Author(s), under exclusive license to Springer Nature Switzerland AG 2025

N. Stock, N. Peim, *The Lacanian Teacher*, The Palgrave Lacan Series, https://doi.org/10.1007/978-3-031-93018-8

practice any unravelling of the chained Borromean knot must entail psychosis, an insight that has implications for Lacanian ontology in general.

Castration Not biological, but Symbolic lack in every subject that we sometimes encounter in others or ourselves. All subjects are castrated as they cannot possess the phallus, e.g., total power/knowledge/relations etc. When the teacher misspells a word on the board they might encounter castration. The signifiers is also castrating as it both attempts to speak our desire but also always falls short, thus the classroom is an inherently castrating place.

Cogito Lacan claims that any philosophy or any thinking that proceeds from Descartes's cogito, that places the ego at the centre of consciousness, must be misguided. The 'I think' reflects the certainty of the ego back to the ego in a gesture that Freud's 'promethean discovery' clearly undermines. Lacan redrafts Descartes's formulation in various ways, including 'I think where I am not, therefore I am where I do not think' (E, p. 166). Language indicates the impossibility of the cogito (as fractured) in the difference between the subject of the statement and the subject of the enunciation.

Consciousness The thoughts that are in your head that have the appearance of being your own and being under your control. The perceptions that you have of the world in any given moment that become formulated as thoughts. These seemingly conscious thoughts are, however, not as they appear. For Lacan they are always traced with the unknowable, be that an Imaginary identification, a Symbolic structure, an unconscious desire, an aspect of the horrifying Real, and so on. Consciousness appears to us as agency, but is destabilised by Lacan.

Death drive The death drive, originally proposed by Sabina Spielrein and developed by Freud in *Beyond the Pleasure Principle* has been variously represented by Lacan. The death drive can be a fundamental tendency of the Symbolic order to produce repetition: 'The death instinct is only the mask of the symbolic order' (II, p. 326). By locating the death drive with the symbolic, Lacan associates it with culture so that it 'is not a question of biology' (E, p. 102), and must be distinguished from the biological instinct to return to the inanimate (VII, pp. 211–12). Later, Lacan associated the death drive with drive in general: 'every drive is virtually a death drive' (E, p.848). Every drive pursues its own extinction, involves repetition, and activates jouissance where enjoyment is also a kind of suffering.

Demand A baby crying for milk, it is the needs of a subject that may be satisfied. If a teacher has a deadline, their demand is met by all of the papers being submitted on time. Often this manifests in the subject as a demand for love; the teacher might feel loved by the students when they complete all of the work for them. Demand can be met through the signifier.

Desire Desire emanates from the unconscious, thus cannot be coherently signified. As such our desire always falls short when we speak it, but we become invested in objects that we believe are desirable (see *objet a*). Unlike demand, desire cannot be satisfied. The teacher who desires to change the lives of their students is perhaps speaking an unconscious desire to, for example, be saved themselves. Anything that the subject feels they want (even it is not their own desire) that does not satisfy them when obtaining it is in the realm of desire; when the baby has had enough milk but still wants more, we see desire.

Discourse Lacan tends to use the word discourse, as distinct, say, from 'speech', to emphasize the external, collective, transindividual dimension of language. The Symbolic order can be divided into 'four discourses' that regulate social interactions and identity positions in speech: the discourse of the master, the discourse of the university, the discourse of the hysteric, and the discourse of the analyst. In this book we have not elaborated these discourses but they represent different modalities of speech that position subjects statements in specific ways rather like modes might be said to work in music.

Drive The engine of desire, it is what keeps us keeping on. They do not have an object they seek like desire, but rather aim desire in a direction. Desire's inexhaustibility is in part due to the constant need for satisfaction of the drives, which can be oral, anal, scopic, or invocatory. Classrooms are dominated by voices and images that are attempting to satisfy the drives, but the demand for rankings might be anally driven. Drives seek their own impossible fulfilment or end, thus are always death driven.

Ego In effect, Lacan's reading of Freud disseats the ego as the centre of the subject. For Lacan, the ego is more like an object, a construction formed initially by the specular image of 'self' as unity—formed, then, in meconnaissance. The ego for Lacan is a 'place' where the subject, a product of the Symbolic order, is alienated in an imaginary formation. Lacan claims that the ego is 'structured like a symptom', albeit a 'privileged symptom' and constitutes 'the mental illness of man' (SI, p. 16). Lacan opposed the idea that the aim of psychoanalysis might be to strengthen the ego.

Fantasy Sharing a structure with anxiety, fantasy is the position the subject has in relation to their object of desire, be it dominating it, dominated by it, trying to get it, and so on. It feeds the Imaginary with images and scenes that we can identify with, thus the countless images of teachers in films populate our fantasies of teaching.

Foreclosure is drawn from the Freudian term '*verwerfung*', a defence mechanism different from repression, that carries an implication of repudiation although for Lacan the thing or idea to be excluded is refused, unacknowledged, unseen, in advance. So foreclosure is distinguished from repression and negation. The foreclosed element remains outside of the structure of the subject. Used in clinical terms to make sense of psychosis, foreclosure can be a useful term in addressing what the Symbolic order may have already failed to acknowledge, to identify what is beyond the ken of consciousness and what may be dangerous to the order of things.

Gaze To do with seeing and being seen, the gaze is a partial object—something that acts as an object that we find desirable but that cannot be found in a material form. The gaze implies not just looking at something or being seen by another, but rather how they work in a larger view: I the teacher see you the student seeing me. My conscious outlook of the world is always coloured by what I unconsciously believe is perceiving me, and how I think I am seen.

Id Lacan's take on the id stresses that the source of its strangeness to the ego is not to be found in hidden instinctual forces, but is essentially linguistic: 'made of the signfier' (IV, p. 49). The id is the unconscious origin of speech, and as such represents the other within. Lacan's rewriting of subjectivity frequently resorts to expressing the idea of the id as an independent, external identity that 'speaks' the subject. Hence the common trope that Lacan claims that languages uses me more than I use language.

Imaginary In Lacan's three registers, the Imaginary is the realm of identification. The labelling of things as signifiers is Imaginary, as this naming gives the illusory impression that we know those things wholly. We also identify with others, thinking that they are what we are like. In this identification, the world of images and appearances comes to constitute our vision of ourselves. When I say I am a teacher, I identify with this Imaginary thing and bring all the associations I have of it with me.

Jouissance Explained in detail in the book, jouissance is literally orgasm, but really entails a realm of pleasure that goes beyond the merely pleasurable into something that might be painful or anxiety inducing.

Lack is related to desire. The Lacanian subject is predicated on lack mobilizing desire. For Lacan this condition is the outcome of language that 'hollows being'. Entry into language, that confers a position in the Symbolic order demands that the subject accept 'castration' that symbolizes the condition of lack. Lack is sometimes understood as the lack of an object, the object of desire, although the object 'itself' remains obscure and may be metonymically deferred along a signifying chain. Lack can, then, be understood as the missing signifier that never arrives. There is no end to lack. Thus lack is related to the death-drive or drive as illustrated in 'fort-da'.

Master signifier The start of a signifying chain that propels meaning to take place. When a teacher starts the lesson with a question like 'What is suffering?', 'suffering' becomes a signifier that will link to other signifiers in continual deferral (until stopped by the point de capiton). Master signifiers are usually the 'big' conceptual worlds that we revolve a lot of our thinking and doing around, some of which might be words like 'education', 'justice', and so on.

Meconnaissance is the condition of subject formation and identity. The subject misrecognizes herself in the position assigned by the symbolic order in language. There is no reaching back to any recognition of a 'true' self since the self—or ego—is forged in the imaginary identification the subject makes with a position in the symbolic order. So the ego is always already an illusory identification with a unified self that has never existed but that may appear to the subject as an equivocal possibility. Louis Althusser famously used Lacan's thinking of meconnaissance to produce the idea of 'interpellation' whereby the social subject is 'hailed' as a certain identity and responds thus assuming that identity.

Metaphor/metonymy For Lacan, metonymy is the movement from one signifier to another along a chain that is hypothetically endless. In language, one thing leads to another. Metonymy is a principle of signification that corresponds with the movement of desire so that, as always with Lacan, the linguistic is intimately bound up with the affective. Metaphor indicates that one thing stands in the place of and for another thing and is in one important sense a condition of language, as metaphor works by substitution. It is easy to see that metaphor and metonymy, sometimes referred to as twin poles of language, are very closely related.

Mirror stage A formative event that is both literal and metaphorical, where the subject believes they encounter themselves as whole. In the image they see in the mirror, which does not have to be a mirror but can be a story, another person, etc., they believe they possess total mastery over themselves. The stage is thus essential in the formation of the ego-ideal, see in the positioning of a teacher in front of a class. The teacher stands as a reflection of the students who has mastered knowledge.

Nachträglichkeit Also known as retroactivity/afterwardsness. The process by which meaning is made in a backwards direction. For example, when asking students to open their books, there is an absence of meaning in terms of which page, which book, actually or metaphorically? This meaning is only affirmed when the sentence finishes with 'to page 43', as only their text book has page numbers. This also works in terms of activation of trauma and primal scenes, which are given weight only when they are encountered again in a different repeated form, rather than when they originally take place.

Nom-du-pere (name of the father/the non-duped-err) In 'rewriting' the Oedipus complex, Lacan refers to the nom-du-pere as a way of insisting on the function of the Symbolic father. We stick to the French in the inscription nom-du-pere as a way of retaining the echo of the 'non' as an interdiction. For Lacan, the father operates as a signifier of an ideal symbolic figure that also represents the law and its prohibition, specifically the prohibition of incest, but metonymically, prohibition in general. In Lacan's mapping of the subject the nom-du-pere is an essential component in the subject's restless accommodation to the order of things, the Symbolic order.

Objet petit a Also know as object a or just 'a'. It is the object cause of desire. As desire is unconscious, an unknowable wish that is tied to our idiosyncrasies, it must find things in the Symbolic to attach to. These thing are just signifiers and therefore cannot be fully obtained, but when we think we get them, they are disappointing as the object of desire from the unconscious has not been realised. Desire will then defer to a new objet a, perhaps one that is metaphorically/metonymically linked to the last one. There is also something *about* the signifier that *causes* it to become desirable, some quality that charms us.

Other/other In simple terms, the other designates what is not the subject, although 'other' is probably among the most complex of Lacanian terms. The little other is distinguished from the big other that signifies something akin to the symbolic order, the ruling order or the injunction that comes form external (to the subject) forces. At the same time, the other is the figure that stands in relation to the subject and that may appear in the (false) guise of completeness, reinforcing the subject's sense of their own castration (incompleteness). In addition, the other may simply signify the other sex that, roughly following Hegel, in its perceived difference offers a shaky sexed identity to the subject.

Phallus Importantly *not* penis though of course linked to it. The phallus is a signifier *of* the lack, in, that it represents wholeness, or lack of lack. It is deliberately masculine in its reference to the patriarchal structure of our world, and is a symbol of power in its refusal to be abolished. It also represents a form of relationality in its interlocking with others. Teachers might present themselves as holding the phallus in being knowledgeable, or believe they have a phallic relationship with students by being able to pass that knowledge onto them—both of which are prone to castration.

Point de capiton The punctuation of a signifying chain. Translatable as 'button tie' or 'quilting point', it indicates the fastening of meaning in language. When a teacher explains a topic that has no meaning to students whatsoever, the *point de capiton* might be a final statement that returns it back to the syllabus. It is also found in educational logics in the Symbolic, for example the end point of education for students.

Primal Scene Freud's patients often uncovered an early traumatic memory that was the core of their symptoms, but it quickly became clear that these memories did not need to be real to have that effect. As such, the primal scene can be any repressed fantasy that results in a behaviour or symptom.

Real In Lacan, the Real is one of three intersecting, overlapping orders of being along with the Symbolic and the Imaginary. The Real is what lies beyond: it is the brute stuff of being beyond symbolization, frightening, formless and unknowable, but nevertheless implacably there. Groping in the dark, we may get some sense of the shapeless noumenal existence of things in the world divested of our systems of meaning and our fantasies of identity. The Real lurks and sometimes intrudes in its utter indifference to our ideas and desires, rather like the iceberg that crashes into the glittering world of the Titanic or the planet Melancholia.

Sign Fundamental to Lacan is the redescription of the sign, classically described by de Saussure as the signifier and signified in a corresponding relationship. Lacan came to insist that the unity of the sign was illusory and that the signified could not be understood as a stable, singular or predictable entity. What Lacan referred to as the sliding of the signified indicated that a sign could only point towards something in a way that must demand an arbitrary point of resolution, so that meaning is always in play and always subject to interpretation.

Signification In Lacan, signification refers to the relation between signifier and signified. Given the priority of the signifier and the elusive quality of the signified the relation is radically mobile so that signification is always a process rather than a decisive event. What's more signification is 'metonymic': in other words, it is interminable, as one signifier activates other signifiers and there is no determinable point the process can end at. Lacan opposes signification to meaning as the latter may imply termination. Signification is to be associated with the imaginary, meaning with the Symbolic.

Signified The signified endlessly slides under the signifier, as Lacan modifies the de Saussurian model of the sign that claims signifier and signified form a unity. For Lacan, the signified—signifying meaning—is endlessly deferred in a movement that corresponds with the obscurely driven mobility of desire. In an obvious sense there is no fixed link between signifier and signified, although the Symbolic order may seek to stabilize that relation into determinate meaning.

Signifier In Ferdinand de Saussure's account of the sign, the signifier is the material component of the sign that points towards a meaning or 'semantic' or conceptual component. De Saussure saw these two components of the sign as being in a close and necessary relation as with two sides of the same coin. For Lacan, however, the sign is, like the subject, barred. The signifier's relation to the signified is enigmatic. The signifieds identity is nebulous and can only be identified by referring again to signifiers. For Lacan it is signfiers that are the basic unit of language rather than signs.

Subject ($) The individual as person, but drawing on the Cartesian figure of the subject as an agent of knowing. Lacan writes the subject as a barred S to imply there *is* a subject, but it is not whole in the way philosophy has made it appear. This lack of wholeness is what constitutes us as a subject of lack, constantly seeking its filling through the mode of desire. There are lots of types of subjects, for example neurotic, psychotic, and also teacher, student, manager.

Subject supposed to know The subject (S.s.S.) who appears to know the answer to another subject's lack. They appear in the clinical setting and the classroom as the all-knowing one who can answer any question we might have. Usually this figure is needed to substantiate the clinical and pedagogical relationship, as one comes to the subject supposed to know looking for answers. Eventually the S.s.S. will reveal themselves as a fraud.

Superego For Lacan, the super-ego takes on the function of an interdiction in the resolution of the Oedipus complex. The super-ego comes to act then as a kind of law, but curiously in line with modern theories of legality, the law is founded in a blind violence of prohibition. The superego is mostly associated in Lacan's psychic ontology with the Symbolic and is to be distinguished from the function and form of the ego ideal that belongs to the Imaginary. The superego's 'unconscious censorship' (E, p.106) is referred to by Lacan as forming a function similar to the Freudian conception of the superego that acts as a dictatorial prohibitor in the regulation of the subject's desire. Later, the super-ego in its imperial role demands enjoyment, being both the instigator of the jouissance it simultaneously prohibits. The strictness of the super-ego becomes a channel for jouissance: expressing a severe command that comes from a place experienced as the will of the Other.

Symbolic Another of Lacan's three registers, the Symbolic is the order of the world that we find ourselves in. It is a cloaking of the Real through language (signifiers), that are linked together as language always is—through grammatical structure. Each little world we find ourselves in is an aspect of the Symbolic, particularly the world of the school for example. But it is always part of a bigger structure—that of education, say.

Topology Lacan's interest in topology, as a psychoanalytic term, seems to have derived from an insistence that the subject of the unconscious can be represented as a bag or a sphere, having an inside and an outside. A far-reaching implication of Lacanian rethinking is that what appears to be naturally determinable as interior, or intimate, is always radically foreign or exterior. Lacan's early description of the unconscious as the discourse of the other correspondingly seems to confound the inside/outside logic, hence Lacan's fascination in the Mobius strip and some of its topological variations like the Klein bottle. It is clear that in Lacan's complicated interest in topology there is the realization of a mathematical mode of figuration for the barred subject, the subject of the signifier as no longer conceivable as interior to itself.

Transference The conversation that takes place unconsciously in any relationship that involves a subject supposed to know and an other. Though we might feel like what we are saying as a teacher about a text is being heard, there will be other messages being communicated via our unconscious that go to the student's unconscious. They might be, for example, you are the child I once was, who I miss and thus will punish you.

Unconscious Lacan emphasises the originality of Freud's 'promethean discovery' of the unconscious. The word unconscious gets used as both adjective and noun by Lacan. For Lacan, the unconscious is primarily linguistic, hence the famous formulation that 'the unconscious is structured like a language'. For Lacan the unconscious is the effects of the signifier on the subject and as such cannot be envisaged as an interior entity. It is transindividual as it is constituted in language that determines the subject via the symbolic order. The unconscious is also a form of memory—a symbolic history. The unconscious is ever-present or ever-active, informing speech and thought obscurely in relation to both desire and repetition.

References

Jacque Lacan's Seminars and Writings

BW Lacan, J. (2017). *Talking to Brick Walls: A Series of Presentations in the Chapel at The Sainte—Anne Hospital* (A. R. Price, Trans.). Polity Press.

E Lacan, J. (2006). *Écrits* (B. Fink, Trans.). W.W. Norton and Co.

FA Lacan, J. (1964). *The Founding Act.* 21st June. lacaninireland.com

I Lacan, J. (1988). *The Seminar: Book I. Freud's Papers on Technique, 1953–54* (J. Forrester, Trans.). Norton.

II Lacan, J. (1988). *The Seminar of Jacques Lacan: Book III. The Ego in Freud's Theory and in the Technique of Psychoanalysis 1954–1955*. Cambridge University Press.

III Lacan, J. (1993). *The Psychoses: The Seminars of Jacque Lacan. Book III* (R. Grigg, Trans.). Routledge.

LT Lacan, J. (1974). *La Troisième, VIIème congrès de l'École freudienne de Paris, Rome.* http://www.valas.fr/IMG/pdf/la_troisieme_integrale.pdf

MT Lacan, J. (2008). *My Teaching.* Verso.

VII Lacan, J. (2008). *The Ethics of Psychoanalysis. The Seminars of Jacques Lacan: Book VII.* Routledge.

VIII Lacan, J. (2017). *Transference. The Seminars of Jacques Lacan: Book VIII.* Polity.

X Lacan, J. (2014). *Anxiety. The Seminars of Jacques Lacan: Book X.* Polity.

XI Lacan, J. (1994). *The Four Fundamental Concepts of Psychoanalysis. The Seminars of Jacques Lacan: Book XI.* Penguin.

XVI Lacan, J. (2024). *From and Other to the Other. The Seminars of Jacques Lacan: Book XVI* (B. Fink, Trans.). Polity.

© The Author(s), under exclusive license to Springer Nature Switzerland AG 2025

N. Stock, N. Peim, *The Lacanian Teacher*, The Palgrave Lacan Series, https://doi.org/10.1007/978-3-031-93018-8

XVII Lacan, J. (2006). *The Other Side of Psychoanalysis: The Seminar of Jacques Lacan: Book XVII* (R. Grigg, Trans.). Norton.

XX Lacan, J. (1999). *On Feminine Sexuality. The Limits of Love and Knowledge. Encore. The Seminar of Jacques Lacan. Book XX.* (B. Fink, Trans.). WW Norton and Co.

XXIII Lacan, J. (2018). *The Sinthome. The Seminar of Jacques Lacan. Book XXIII.* Polity.

Freud Standard Edition

SE II Freud, S. (1895). *The Standard Edition of the Complete Psychological Works of Sigmund Freud, Volume II (1893–1895): Studies on Hysteria.* The Hogarth Press.

SE VII Freud, S. (1895). *The Standard Edition of the Complete Psychological Works of Sigmund Freud, Volume II (1893–1895): Studies on Hysteria.* The Hogarth Press.

SE XI Freud, S. (1910). *Five Lectures on Psycho-Analysis, Leonardo da Vinci and Other Works. The Standard Edition of the Complete Psychological Works of Sigmund Freud.* The Hogarth Press.

SE XII Freud, S. (1913). *The Standard Edition of the Complete Psychological Works of Sigmund Freud, Volume XII (1911–1913): The Case of Schreber, Papers on Technique and Other Works. The Standard Edition of the Complete Psychological Works of Sigmund Freud.* The Hogarth Press.

SE XIII Freud, S. (1913). *The Standard Edition of the Complete Psychological Works of Sigmund Freud, Volume XIII.* The Hogarth Press.

SE XIV Freud, S. (1915). *The Unconscious. The Standard Edition of the Complete Psychological Works of Sigmund Freud, 14.* Hogarth.

SE XIX Freud, S. (1923). *The Ego and the Id. The Standard Edition of the Complete Psychological Works of Sigmund Freud, Volume XIX (1923–1925).* The Hogarth Press.

SE XV Freud, S. (1916). *Introductory Lectures on Psycho-Analysis. The Standard Edition of the Complete Psychological Works of Sigmund Freud* 15. The Hogarth Press.

SE XVIII Freud, S. (1922). *Beyond the Pleasure Principle, Group Psychology and Other Works. The Standard Edition of the Complete Psychological Works of Sigmund Freud 18.* The Hogarth Press.

SE XXI Freud, S. (1930). *Civilization and Its Discontents. The Standard Edition of the Complete Psychological Works of Sigmund Freud, Volume XXI (1927–1931): The Future of an Illusion, Civilization and Its Discontents, and Other Works* (pp. 57–146). The Hogarth Press.

Index[1]

A
Alienation, 39, 166–168, 167n1, 173
Althusser, Luis, 15n5, 50, 86
Anxiety, 8, 14, 48, 51, 58, 58n2, 62, 89, 103, 104, 111, 118, 130, 138, 141, 148, 150
Architecture
of classroom, 17, 19, 46, 95
of playground, 17, 19
of school, 17
Assessment, 4n1, 14, 21, 39–41, 60, 80, 86, 107, 109, 115, 118n9, 119, 120, 150, 173, 179
Authoritarianism, 67, 106, 129, 148, 154

B
Bar, *see* Split subject
Barthes, Roland, 71, 96, 108, 149, 164, 165, 172, 174
Bartleby, 160–164
Beckett, Samuel, 89, 166, 166–167n1
Being, 10–15, 12n3, 15n5, 18, 43, 50, 75, 80, 103, 106n3, 112, 116, 157
Bernstein, Basil, 24, 39, 40, 43, 99–101, 107, 109, 110
Bourdieu, Pierre, 24, 86
Brecht, Bertolt, 97, 166–168, 166–167n1
Britzman, Deborah, 5, 7, 41, 42, 47, 50, 52, 57, 61, 69, 76, 77, 99, 131, 132, 138, 142, 154, 165, 166, 169

C
Cartel, 4, 36–37
Castration, 73, 100, 104, 132, 160
Cioran, Emil, 10, 81, 101, 160, 166
Clinic, 111, 117, 128, 173

[1] Note: Page numbers followed by 'n' refer to notes.

© The Author(s), under exclusive license to Springer Nature Switzerland AG 2025

N. Stock, N. Peim, *The Lacanian Teacher*, The Palgrave Lacan Series, https://doi.org/10.1007/978-3-031-93018-8

Clown, *see* Fool
Cogito, 12
Comedy, 80, 168
Consciousness, 12, 13, 105, 128, 129, 131, 133, 137, 140, 143, 182
  as *conscientização*, 128
Curriculum, 3, 13, 16, 18, 20, 24, 35, 39, 50, 52, 66, 70, 71, 76, 77, 80, 82, 86, 87, 98, 109, 110, 116, 118–119n9, 122, 152, 171, 173, 177

D

Death drive, 2, 6, 8, 114, 135–137, 135n2, 162–164, 182–184
Demand, 31–33, 34n2, 39, 42, 44, 46, 48, 50, 51, 66, 68n3, 72, 77, 78, 82–86, 88, 96, 101–103, 112, 113n7, 118, 131, 142, 148, 151, 155, 157, 159, 162, 163, 166, 167n1, 171, 172, 174–176, 180–183
Department for Education (DfE), 56n1, 59, 60, 63, 67, 69, 70, 77, 116, 119n9, 120, 121, 148
Derrida, Jacques, 7, 22, 23, 34n2, 43, 71, 80, 87, 97n2, 111, 120, 134, 163, 176–180
Desire
  of the Other, 14, 31, 35, 44, 48, 65, 76, 163, 183
  pedagogy of, 105, 110, 123, 137–139, 155, 171, 182
  teacher's, 2, 35, 48, 56, 57, 59, 79, 154, 171, 181
Disavowal, 94, 136
Discourse
  of the master, 106, 106n3
  of the university, 36n3, 106, 107, 110
Drive, 2, 6, 8, 41, 44, 58, 67, 72, 75, 114, 131, 135–137, 135n2, 149, 156, 159, 162–164, 171, 182–184

E

Ego
  destitution, 47, 58
  ego-ideal/ideal-ego, 45, 48–50, 52, 56, 59–61, 75, 77n5, 88, 89, 95, 119, 130, 166, 167, 171
English
  curriculum, 70, 71, 82, 86, 87, 110
  literature, 2, 3, 70, 83
Enjoyment, *see* Jouissance
Ethics, 40, 44, 65, 74, 75n4, 76, 77, 85, 89, 101, 108, 115n8, 123, 132, 155, 157, 159, 164
Examination, *see* Assessment

F

Fantasy, 2–5, 9, 15, 19, 20, 23, 25, 30, 32, 37, 40, 46–48, 52, 56–89, 94, 97, 99, 103, 112, 115n8, 117, 119, 119n9, 120, 128–132, 141, 142, 148, 151, 152, 154, 159, 180, 183, 184
Felman, Shoshana, 4n1, 5–7, 30, 50, 52, 111, 117, 138, 164
Films/television
  Another Round, 64
  Dangerous Minds, 18, 20, 23, 62, 65, 70
  Dead Poets Society, 23, 50, 62, 70
  Detachment, 22, 67, 70, 71
  DfE, 63, 67
  Donnie Darko, 70, 120
  Half Nelson, 19, 62, 63, 120, 166
  Monsieur Lazhar, 66, 70, 181

The Ron Clark Story, 33, 62, 65, 151
Teachers, 63, 70
Whiplash, 72–74, 120
Fool, 80–82, 96, 167, 168, 171
Foreclosure, 75
Foucault, Michel, 7, 45, 87, 101, 114, 123
Freire, Paulo, 128–134, 136
Freud, Sigmund, 6–11, 13, 15n5, 36, 40, 43, 44, 50, 57, 87, 88, 94, 95n1, 104, 111, 114, 116, 117, 133, 135, 135n2, 136, 138, 141, 149, 150, 155, 158, 162, 168, 179–181

G
Gaze, 16, 18, 19, 45–49, 77, 95, 99, 118n9, 130, 166n1, 167, 169, 174

H
Heidegger, Martin, 7, 10, 11, 13, 14, 22n7, 40, 43, 157, 158
Hysteria, 9, 179, 182

I
Id, 43
Identification
imaginary, 15, 17, 20, 25, 35, 40, 48, 81, 82, 107, 139
misidentification/*méconnai ssance*, 40
Ignorance, 9, 31, 32, 34, 36, 52, 139, 142

J
Jouissance, 2
Other, 153, 155, 181, 184
phallic, 104
sadomasochistic, 184
signifier of, 7, 72, 102, 139, 140, 155, 159, 170, 172, 173, 175, 176
Joyce, James, 81, 83, 106, 175, 176, 179, 180

K
Knowledge, 3, 5, 6, 9, 11–13, 15, 16, 18n6, 24, 25, 31–34, 36, 39, 40, 42, 46, 51, 52, 59, 60, 62, 65, 66, 68–71, 73, 78n6, 79, 82, 84, 87, 100, 101, 103–120, 108n4, 113n7, 115n8, 128, 130, 132–134, 138–143, 152, 153, 157, 172, 180–183

L
Lack, 32, 41, 44, 47, 70, 89, 101, 104–118, 128–132, 139–143, 149, 150, 154, 155, 159, 160, 162, 171, 177, 178, 181, 182
Law, 38, 43, 48, 96, 113n7, 149, 151, 152, 155, 159, 160, 163–167, 172, 174, 182, 184
of classroom, 151, 152, 159, 172, 174, 182, 184
Letter, 35, 50, 69, 168–172
Literature, *see* English

M
Malabou, Catherine, 8, 87, 132–136, 157, 162, 184
Masochism, 47, 73, 148, 153
  See also Sadism, sadomasochism
Master, 5, 32, 41, 43, 60, 73, 76, 98, 103, 105, 106, 106n3, 110, 115, 128, 129, 131, 133, 150, 155, 159, 161, 163, 165, 167, 171, 174, 181, 182
  mastery, 5, 14, 33, 43, 70, 72, 73, 83, 87, 103, 111, 112, 117, 118, 140, 157, 194
  signifier, 41, 60, 76, 98, 105, 110, 128, 131, 159, 165, 174, 193
Memory
  storage system, 116, 117
  wunderblock, 117
Metaphor, 69, 79, 101, 102, 116, 169, 180
Metonymy, 79
Mirror Stage, 45, 47, 48, 58, 64, 94, 95, 99

N
Nachträglichkeit, 59, 82
Neoliberalism, 44, 98, 151, 152
Nietzsche, Friedrich, 156, 158, 165
Nom-du-pere/name of the father/the non-duped-err, *see* Paternal

O
Objet a, 35, 58n2, 60, 72, 88, 98, 119n9, 128, 169–171, 174, 178
Observation, 18, 32, 51, 60, 77, 148, 174
Ofsted, 56n1, 60, 61, 70, 152
Ontology, 10–25, 12n3, 30, 38, 61, 74, 75, 75n4, 157, 158
Other
  big Other, 15, 38, 39, 42, 44, 48, 49, 69, 72–74, 77, 96, 98, 105, 106n3, 139, 153, 155, 156, 160, 165, 166, 173, 182, 184
  as education, 38, 39, 48, 76, 106n3, 119, 139, 173, 183, 184
  as student, 30, 31, 65, 97, 170, 171, 183, 184

P
Paradigm, 3, 7, 11, 30, 112–114, 115n8, 116, 133, 149
Paternal, 68, 174, 175
Pedagogy
  anti-, 138, 139
  critical, 5, 6, 8, 101, 129–134, 137, 139, 141, 182
  does not exist, 98, 129
  liberatory, 8, 38, 98, 128–134, 155, 183
  mundane, 100, 128
  pedagogical relationship, 98, 101, 119, 128, 129, 131, 136, 138–143, 148–149
  psychological, 100
Pessimism, 10, 135, 143, 166
Phallus, 104, 105, 140
  phallic stage, 94
Piaget, Jean, 46, 99, 100
Plasticity, 134–136, 136n3, 157, 162
Point de capiton, 118–123
Progress, 15, 16, 21, 24, 39, 60, 87, 89, 99, 100, 111, 114,

118, 120, 121, 123, 152, 156, 181, 182
Psychology
  developmental, 116
  and education, 99

R
Racism, 154
Real, 12–14, 17, 20–25, 30, 35, 38, 42, 43, 52, 57, 58, 66, 69, 76, 79, 86, 87, 96, 100, 104, 112, 112n6, 114, 129, 132, 134, 137, 138, 141, 156–159, 162, 166n1, 171, 174, 180, 182
Repetition, 25, 31, 39, 73, 150, 173
  compulsion to repeat, 150
Reshe, Julie, 33, 34, 34n1, 128, 131, 134–137, 136n3, 143, 157, 162–164, 168, 184
Retroactivity, *see Nachträglichkeit*

S
Sade, Marquis de, 58n2, 73, 74
Sadism, 73, 148
  sadomasochism, 154
School/schooling, 2–6, 8, 13, 17, 19, 20, 22–25, 22n7, 30, 34, 36–38, 40, 42–44, 47, 50, 56, 58n2, 60, 61, 63, 66, 67, 69–71, 77–79, 78n6, 82, 83, 85, 94–96, 98, 106, 109, 110, 118n9, 120, 122, 128, 129, 132n1, 133, 134, 139, 148, 150–152, 154, 155, 162, 164–168, 177
  deschooling, 8, 37, 128
  of thought, 36
  See also Architecture
Science, 5, 11, 14, 100, 111–116, 115n8, 135
Sexuation, 98, 139, 140, 155
Shakespeare, William, 2, 80, 101, 103, 108
Signifier
  binary, 39
  of lack, 104–118, 128–132, 139–142, 149, 154, 155, 159, 160, 171, 182 (*see also* Phallus)
  signifying chain, 34, 41, 43, 121, 168, 175
Speech
  as blahblahblah, 176, 179, 180, 182
  as lalangue, 175, 178
Split subject, 6, 8, 43, 66, 84, 98, 102, 133
Stage
  anal, 103, 149, 191
  oral, 94
  phallic, 94
  school, 95
  theatrical, 95
Subject
  split, 11, 39, 43
  supposed to know/S.s.S, 50–52, 117, 118, 129, 171
Superego, 77n5, 162
Symbolic, 3–5, 9, 12–18, 18n6, 20–25, 30, 35, 38–43, 46, 48–51, 57, 60, 65, 68n3, 72, 73, 75, 78, 79, 81, 83–85, 89, 94–96, 98–100, 104, 105, 109, 110, 112, 114–116, 119–123, 128–130, 132–135, 137, 138, 140, 142, 149–152, 154, 156–159, 161–164, 166, 167, 171–176, 178–182
Symptom, 34, 162, 179, 180

T
Teacher
standards, 24, 56, 56n1, 70
trainee teacher, 10, 61, 64, 77, 121Topology, 12n3, 78, 97n2
Tragedy
Antigone, 155, 156
Attic, 156, 157
Birth of, 156
A Doll's House, 155
Hamlet, 155, 156
Oedipus, 156
Tragic fool, 80, 82, 96, 168, 171
Transference, 52, 137, 141, 142, 168–170
Truth, 13, 65, 87, 108, 109, 112–114, 118, 158, 163, 169, 170, 172, 180, 181

U
Unconscious, 3, 6, 8, 9, 12, 14, 15, 19, 22, 35, 42–45, 51, 52, 58, 67, 79, 98–100, 103, 111, 113, 114, 117, 120, 132, 137, 139, 141, 142, 148, 150, 157, 170, 179–182

V
Viva voce, 25
Vygotsky, Lev, 18n6, 46, 99, 100

W
Wound, *see* Split subject

Z
Žižek, Slavoj, 48, 49, 74, 160, 161
Zupančič, Alenka, 10, 156, 157, 159, 168

The manufacturer's authorised representative in the EU is Springer Nature Customer Service Centre GmbH, Europaplatz 3, 69115 Heidelberg, Germany. If you have any concerns regarding our products, please contact ProductSafety@springernature.com

Printed and bound by CPI Group (UK) Ltd, Croydon, CR0 4YY
30/09/2026
02225583-0004